WHY Can't I KEEP UP Anymore?

WHY Can't I KEEP UP Anymore?

A GUIDE TO REGAINING ENERGY, FOCUS AND PEAK PHYSICAL & SEXUAL PERFORMANCE FOR Men Over 40

Deborah Matthew, MD
Best-selling author of *"This is NOT Normal!"*

Optimal Wellness Press

Copyright ©2020 by Deborah Matthew, MD

All rights reserved. No part of this book may be reproduced or transmitted in any form or by any means without written permission of the publisher, except in the case of brief quotations embodied in critical articles and reviews.

This material has been written and published solely for educational purposes. The author and the publisher shall have neither liability nor responsibility to any person or entity with respect to any loss, damage, or injury caused or alleged to be caused directly or indirectly by the information contained in this book.

The author of this book does not dispense medical advice or prescribe the use of any technique as a form of treatment for physical, emotional, or medical problems without the advice of a qualified healthcare provider, either directly or indirectly. The intent of the author is only to offer information of a general nature to help you in your quest for well-being. In the event you use any of the information in this book for yourself or others, which is your constitutional right, the author and the publisher assume no responsibility for your actions.

Statements made in this book have not been evaluated by the Food and Drug Administration. This book and its contents are not intended to diagnose, treat, or cure any infection, injury, or illness, or prevent any disease. Results vary and each person's experience is unique.

Published by Optimal Wellness Press

ISBN (paperback): 978-0-578-78394-9
ISBN (ebook): 978-0-578-78394-9

Cover and interior design by Christy Collins, Constellation Book Services

Printed in the United States of America

To my patients, who inspire me to always keep learning.

Acknowledgments

It turns out that writing a book isn't the hardest part. Finishing the book and getting it out in the world is the challenge! It would not have been possible without the help, support and creative genius of my husband, Matt. He put up endless requests for "what do you think of this….?" and never complained, so he deserves a lot of credit.

I'm grateful to my team at Signature Wellness - Staci Burrell, Nicole Bentivegna, Marci Cheney, Heather Baerga, Debbie Dalessandro, Margit Magee, Ashley Carpenter, Eleanor Riccardi, Rosalie Natoli, Isabella Natoli, Estelle Davis, and James Chmelik. Your support and collaboration have given me the space to write another book. A special thanks to Nicole for helping with proofreading and offering feedback.

I owe a lot to my mentors. My dad taught me to always keep learning. John Linton and Charles Webb helped me put my practice in order so that I could have the time to write. I wouldn't be where I am today without Clint Arthur, who saw more in me than I could see for myself.

I appreciate the creative wisdom of Cristina Smith and Valerie Cassity. Thanks for your patience and guidance in editing the manuscript. And a special thank you to Christy Collins for the fabulous cover.

Contents

Acknowledgments	*v*
Introduction	*1*
Chapter 1: Why Your Doctor Hasn't Already Helped You	9
Chapter 2: Why Testosterone is Important For Men	15
Chapter 3: How Does Testosterone Work	29
Chapter 4: What Causes Low T?	35
Chapter 5: How to Diagnose Low T	49
Chapter 6: Medical Treatment For Low T	59
Chapter 7: Lifestyle Changes For Optimal Health	85
Chapter 8: Supplements for Men's Health	95
Chapter 9: Stressed Out: Cortisol and Your Health	113
Chapter 10: Five Steps to Stronger Erections	139
Chapter 11: Next Steps	151
Glossary	*159*
References	*169*
About the Author	*177*

Introduction

When you were a teenager, you could probably eat junk food without gaining weight, study for hours and be able to retain lots of information, and stay up all night and still function the next day.

But over time things change.

Your waist may have expanded. Your hairline may have receded. Your erections may not be quite the same. Maybe your doctor has starting to recommend prescriptions for your cholesterol or your blood pressure.

Maybe you just don't feel quite right. Sometimes it can be hard to put your finger on what's changed. I hear a lot of men describe feeling "older". More tired, less focused, less driven. You may notice that your muscle mass has decreased, you're gaining weight, and you don't feel as strong as you used to, but it's hard to muster up the motivation to head to the gym to do something about it. In fact, you may find yourself sitting on the couch mindlessly watching golf, or surfing the net instead of being productive and getting things done.

Men being men, the only thing you are less likely to do than ask for directions when you're lost is head to the doctor. And even if you do, your doctor is unlikely to have the answers. Sure, they have lots of prescriptions—for your cholesterol, your blood pressure, and your blood sugar. They have anti-depressants, antacids, and sleeping pills. Even pills to help you achieve better erections.

Unfortunately, taking the pills may not get you the results that you're looking for. The truth is, the medicines don't really make you WELL—they are mostly just doing damage control and minimizing your symptoms. What happens when you stop taking the drug? Your symptoms will likely just come back. Whatever is causing you to have those symptoms in the first place is still there!

The good news is there are many things you can do to give yourself better odds of staying healthy and feeling good, and we're going to talk about them in this book.

I want to tell you the story of one of my patients (we'll call him Bob).

Bob is an executive in his 50s. He is average height, has brown hair that's starting to gray at the temples, and he has a bit of a spare tire that didn't used to be there. His job is stressful—managing a team to make sure they are meeting their sales goals. He used to be competitive and thrive on stress. In fact, he was one of the top performers in his company. Lately, a lack of focus and motivation have

Introduction

become a problem, and his job feels much more difficult. He is fearful about being replaced and worries that if loses his job he won't be able to provide for his family.

Bob knew he just wasn't keeping up anymore and that something was wrong. He values his health, so every year he goes in for his annual physical. A couple of years ago, he complained about not sleeping well, so his doctor gave him sleeping pills. Last year, when he complained that he didn't feel like himself he was given antidepressants.

This year? His cholesterol was up. And how do you think his doctor handled that? Of course! Now he's supposed to start taking Lipitor too.

On a sunny Thursday afternoon, Bob found himself sitting behind the wheel of his car in the drive-thru lane at his local pharmacy, holding three prescriptions in his hand, thinking, "This doesn't feel right. I'm doing what they tell me to do—I'm going for my appointments, I'm taking my pills, but they aren't making me any healthier. I just feel older. I've got no drive. I've lost my edge. Where is this going to end up?"

As he's sitting there waiting his turn and watching cars drive by, he thinks to himself "If I was a car, I feel like I'd be an old beater that can barely make it up the hill. But that's not what I want. I want to feel like a finely tuned, high performance sports car!"

Over the last few years, Bob's wife (we'll call her Maryann), had been coming to see me. Bob had watched her lose weight, get her energy back and even have more interest in sex, which was an area that was starting to become a problem for him. While he was feeling older and more worried about his performance, she was looking and feeling younger! So, he decided to come see me.

When he sat down with me in my office, he said, "Dr. Deb—I don't know if I'm going to be able to do all the things you ask me to do. But I know that I've got to try something different, because what I'm doing just isn't working."

We ran a comprehensive lab panel and found that Bob was low in Vitamins D and B12, his inflammation markers were high, cortisol (his stress hormone) was up, and his testosterone level was low. My team and I started him on a nutrition and lifestyle program, with some nutritional supplements based on his lab results.

Within three months, Bob had lost 20 pounds. His cholesterol was normal—without medication. He was off his sleeping pills and antidepressants and he felt great! His energy and memory were improved, his ED was better, and he got his drive back. He was killing it at work and at the end of the quarter he was expecting a great bonus!

Bob feels so good that he's not finding it hard to stick to his improved lifestyle habits. He knows how he felt before, and he doesn't want to go back!

Here's what I've known for years, and what Bob now realizes…

If you want a high performance life, you need to treat yourself like a high performance vehicle. If you drive a Porsche you're not going to put cheap gas in the tank, take

Introduction

it off-roading, or leave it out in a hailstorm. You're going to use premium motor oil and get the engine tuned. Why don't you treat yourself that way?

You only get one body. It is not leased. You can't trade it in. Even the best health insurance policy in the world can't write it off and replace it with a new one.

If you're feeling less like a high performance vehicle and more like a high mileage beater that's scratched and dented with barely enough horsepower to get you to your destination, please know that help is available. The solution is not usually found in the bottom of a prescription bottle and it's not always covered by your health insurance. But you deserve to love the way you feel and to live well. Because living well is the best medicine!

The truth is that while you can't control everything about your health, there is a lot that you can do to improve it! Many people think that their genes determine their health. The truth is that genes only affect 20% of your health. 80% of your health is determined by the decisions you make today—whether to eat some veggies, whether you smoke, how much alcohol you drink, how you're managing stress, whether you're moving your body.

My goal is to help you resolve the root cause of your health issues so you can get well, get off prescription drugs, and love the way you feel!

I believe this is possible, and here's how I got there.

I started my career as a regular MD, and initially I was happy. But my health wasn't the greatest. I was "healthy" in the sense that I didn't have any serious diseases, but things just weren't right.

I was tired ALL the time. I struggled with my weight, and I just didn't feel like myself. My husband and kids noticed the difference, too—I was irritable and flew off the handle over every little thing. In fact, my husband started calling me from the car on his way home from work. He could tell by the tone of my voice whether it was a good day or not, and whether he should put on a suit of armor for his own protection before he walked in the door.

I didn't mean to be the "Wicked Witch of the West." I didn't want to always be shrieking at my kids or aggravated with my husband. I knew that how I was feeling was NOT normal. It was so confusing because nothing in my medical training helped me understand why I was feeling this way. I wasn't really depressed, I was just kind of worn out and mean. And I didn't have any idea what to do about it.

My quest to solve my own issues led to my discovery of Functional Medicine. This is a different way of thinking about your health. Practitioners of Functional Medicine will evaluate your body and see which parts are functioning well, and which parts aren't so great—then get to work fixing those things! Natural treatments are used whenever possible, and prescription medicines are saved as a last resort.

This is quite different than what we learn at medical school. We are taught to ask the question WHAT? What is the diagnosis? For example insomnia, anxiety, or high cholesterol. And then we ask, what is the best drug to treat this with?

Introduction

In Functional Medicine, we spend more time asking the question WHY? Why was I irritable all the time? Why has your cholesterol started to go up? (Hint: it isn't a Lipitor deficiency...)

Instead of just treating your symptoms with drugs, which often just put a Band-Aid on your symptoms and don't really make you well, we look for the ROOT CAUSES of your health issues, and then work with you to resolve them.

Instead of taking anxiety pills or antidepressants, I had my hormone and vitamin levels measured and looked at markers of inflammation and other factors that affect energy, mood, and metabolism. It turns out I had problems with hormone imbalances and some nutritional deficiencies. Once those issues were corrected, I went back to feeling like my old self again! I got my energy back, my kids got their mom back, and my husband got his wife back. I got my life back!

But I couldn't go back to practicing medicine the old way, treating everything with my prescription pad. It just didn't make sense anymore.

Over the past 13 years I've helped over 4,000 men and women get well, regain their energy, and live life to the fullest. And I love what I do.

I am sometimes asked why a woman doctor works with men's health issues. I don't think it is unusual (after all there are a lot of great male gynecologists) and I am really committed to men's health (as I believe most women are). But here's the real story.

Why Can't I Keep Up Anymore?

Initially when I started my practice I worked mostly with women. Once my female patients got their energy and sex drive back, they started asking if I could work with their husbands. They felt great, but their husbands couldn't keep up with them...so I started working with more and more men!

If you know that you're not quite keeping up anymore—if you're feeling "old", more irritable, foggy brained, achy, or just not as good as you think you could feel—please know that help is available! You do not have to put up with feeling this way.

Let's get started by talking about how you can take control of your health! I'll be sharing tips on how to:

- Help your brain perform at an optimal level
- Keep your body healthy and pain-free
- Restore sexual performance
- Feel great!

You deserve to live well.
I believe living well is the best medicine!

CHAPTER 1

Why Your Doctor Hasn't Already Helped You

Do you think that Americans are the healthiest people in the world?

Not only are we not, but we fall embarrassingly low on the list. According to the 2019 Bloomberg Global Health Index, Spain is the healthiest country in the world, closely followed by Italy, Iceland, and Japan. The US was ranked way down at #35, below countries like Costa Rica, Croatia, and Cuba. To come up with the scores, they looked at factors like:

- Health risks (tobacco use, high blood pressure, obesity)
- Availability of clean water
- Life expectancy
- Malnutrition
- Causes of death

Why Can't I Keep Up Anymore?

I would go so far as to say that I believe we have a health crisis in America. Do you agree?

Despite our not-so-great health, we have the most expensive healthcare system in the world!

We spend WAY more money per person than any other developed country. Since we're spending so much money, you'd expect that we should have the healthiest people. Doesn't that make sense? If you have the most expensive car in the world, wouldn't you expect it be the fastest, most comfortable, most technologically advanced vehicle? Otherwise, wouldn't you be mad that you didn't get your money's worth?

We're spending a lot, but where is all of that money going? The pharmaceutical industry, insurance companies, and large hospital systems are profiting, but it doesn't seem that the average American is coming out ahead.

I would argue that even if every man, woman, and child had fabulous health insurance (don't hold your breath on this one, but just pretend with me for a minute) we still wouldn't fix the problem, because I believe we're not providing the RIGHT medical care.

Here's the problem: In America, we're great at acute care medicine.

If you are injured in a car crash, with broken bones or internal bleeding, we can scoop you up in an ambulance and whisk you into the emergency room in no time flat. A Cracker Jack team of doctors and nurses will patch you up and have you good as new.

Why Your Doctor Hasn't Already Helped You

If you have crushing chest pain because you are in the middle of having a heart attack, we can use the most sophisticated lab tests and medical equipment to figure out exactly where the problem is and how to fix it.

Our modern technology is so impressive! Did you know that we have the capability of doing surgery with robotic instruments, where the doctor and the patient aren't even at the same hospital? It's truly amazing.

But…..most Americans suffer from CHRONIC conditions like cancer, heart disease, arthritis, and diabetes. We have medicines for most of these, but no cures. Unfortunately, our health system doesn't do a great job with chronic conditions.

Many of the medicines we use are just putting Band-Aids on your symptoms or doing "damage control" to try and minimize the complications of your health condition. Medicines can be very important, and sometimes life-saving, but they usually can't make you well. I believe the best option is to do your best to avoid getting sick in the first place!

I don't think the health crisis is your doctor's fault. Your doctor was trained to treat diseases with drugs. They only have 7-15 minutes to talk to you and they are trapped in a system where they are only allowed to do what your insurance will pay for.

Health insurance is part of the problem, so let's talk about it a little more. You may not be thrilled with your health insurance (I'm certainly not thrilled with mine), but you need it. Remember, we have the most expensive health care

Why Can't I Keep Up Anymore?

system in the world! Medical bills are one of the top reasons for bankruptcy in America. In fact, a Harvard study found that 62% of personal bankruptcies are due to medical bills.

I don't know the answers to fix all of our health insurance challenges in this country. But I do want to encourage you to think about your health insurance differently.

Let's think about some of the other insurances that you're familiar with, like your auto insurance and your homeowners policy.

If the paint on your house is peeling, or your carpets are stained, would you expect your homeowners policy to replace them? Of course not—that would be considered routine maintenance, and you would be responsible for that.

If your tires are bald, or your brake pads are worn, would you expect your car insurance to cover these? Once again, this is routine maintenance, and not covered. Now, if you DON'T do the routine maintenance and your brakes fail or your tires blow and you crash your car—then your insurance will kick in!

The truth about your auto insurance and your homeowners policy is that even though you pay it, you hope you never need it. If you do, it means that a tornado blew the roof off your home, or your house burned down or some other terrible thing happened!

I would argue that your health insurance is similar. First of all, it's a misnomer. Kind of like life insurance—which is really death insurance if you think about it. Health insurance is really disease insurance, and you need it. No matter how

Why Your Doctor Hasn't Already Helped You

well you take care of yourself, bad things can happen to good people and if you ever need a kidney transplant or have a severe injury, the medical bills will pile up fast. So, you need to have your health insurance, but don't want to have to use it! Get it?

Do you want to regain your energy, drive and focus? Lose weight? Or just feel like the best version of yourself? If so, you are going to need to take charge of your own health and not rely on your doctor or your health insurance to get you there.

In the next chapters, we'll talk about some of the important factors that may be affecting your current health, such as low testosterone, stress, nutrition and toxins, and I'll give you tips on how you can start turning things around.

CHAPTER 2

Why Testosterone is Important For Men

What qualities do we associate with manhood? Strength, confidence, competitive drive, assertiveness? Testosterone supports all of these.

As a man, when you wake up in the morning and your feet hit the floor, you should feel like you are ready to conquer the world! If instead you feel anxious, nervous, and lack confidence, or if you feel tired, depressed, and "old", there may be a problem.

Your hormones affect who you are on the inside, how you relate to other people, and how you react to the world around you. Testosterone is the primary hormone that we think of in men, although of course you have many different hormones that work together to promote health and well-being.

As you age, your hormone pattern changes. Testosterone levels gradually decrease. It's not as sudden and dramatic as women going through menopause—it's more like a slow,

Why Can't I Keep Up Anymore?

hard to notice decline. Until one day you find yourself sitting on the couch in your underpants watching bowling and wondering, "What happened to me?"

Testosterone and your behavior

There has been quite a lot of research done to look at how testosterone affects behavior in men.

One study looked at stock traders. Traders had their testosterone level checked in the morning, then they were observed on the stock trading floor over the day. They found that the men with higher testosterone levels made the most risky trades, and made the most money. (1)

Another study found that giving male stock traders testosterone to artificially increase their level resulted in the tendency to overestimate future stock values and change their trading behavior, leading to dangerous prices bubbles and subsequent crashes. (2)

Now, I'm not saying that a higher testosterone level will make you rich, but it certainly affects your behavior. If you are in a job that requires motivation and competitive drive, then it's possible that a problem with testosterone could be affecting your job performance (and possibly your income.)

Testosterone has also been shown to decrease the incidence of lying in men. Men were given money based on a roll of dice that they self-reported. They could lie to increase their payout without the chance of being caught. Men who had been given a testosterone injection had lower payouts. While there was lying in both groups, the men with

Why Testosterone is Important for Men

the testosterone were less likely to be dishonest. (3)

Other studies show that testosterone levels are affected by things happening around you.

According to a study done by a graduate student at the University of Utah, after a sports match supporters of the winning team had a 20% boost in testosterone levels, and supporters of the losing team had a 20% dip in testosterone. (4)

Testosterone levels went up after driving a sports car and went down after driving a family sedan. (5)

Men with higher testosterone levels tend to show more of a preference for higher status things, like expensive cars and designer clothes. According to one of the researchers, Colin Camerer of the California Institute of Technology, "In our closest animal kin, males spend a lot of time and energy fighting to establish dominance. We do, too, but our weapons are what we wear, drive, and live in rather than claws, fists, and muscles." (6)

Have you ever fallen in love, and had more energy, been in a better mood, and felt quite different? Part of the explanation is that a new relationship can give you a testosterone boost.

Testosterone and your health

Testosterone plays many roles in your body. It affects your brain, muscles, kidneys, bones, liver, skin, and more. Here is a list of some important things that testosterone does for you:

Why Can't I Keep Up Anymore?

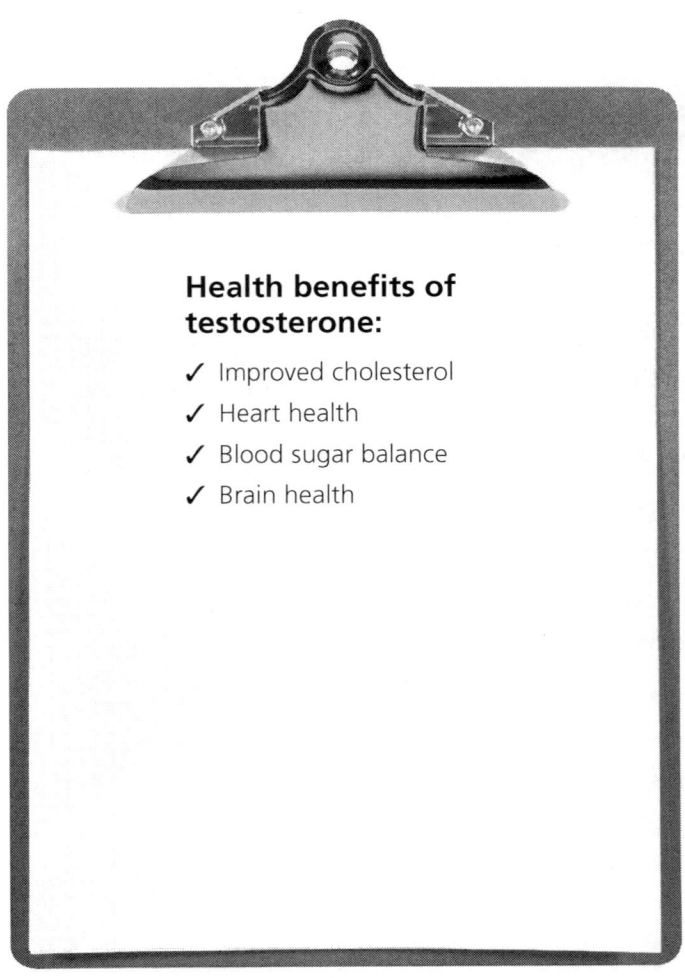

Health benefits of testosterone:

- ✓ Improved cholesterol
- ✓ Heart health
- ✓ Blood sugar balance
- ✓ Brain health

Why Testosterone is Important for Men

Cardiovascular health

Testosterone helps to keep your heart healthy (your heart, after all, is a muscle). There have been many, many research studies done that show how important testosterone is to heart health.

Cholesterol

Testosterone helps maintain normal cholesterol levels. In fact, testosterone is actually made from cholesterol! If you are low in testosterone, one of the ways your body helps to compensate is to make more cholesterol (the building block it needs to make more testosterone). Some men see their cholesterol improve when testosterone levels are restored.

Blood sugar metabolism

Testosterone is very important for normal blood sugar levels. Men with diabetes have a higher risk of having low testosterone, and men with low testosterone have a higher risk of developing diabetes.

Brain health

Testosterone is critical for energy and for sleep. Lack of energy is a common complaint when testosterone levels dip.

Memory

Testosterone helps with memory, focus, and visual-spatial skills. There is an increased risk of Alzheimer's in older

Why Can't I Keep Up Anymore?

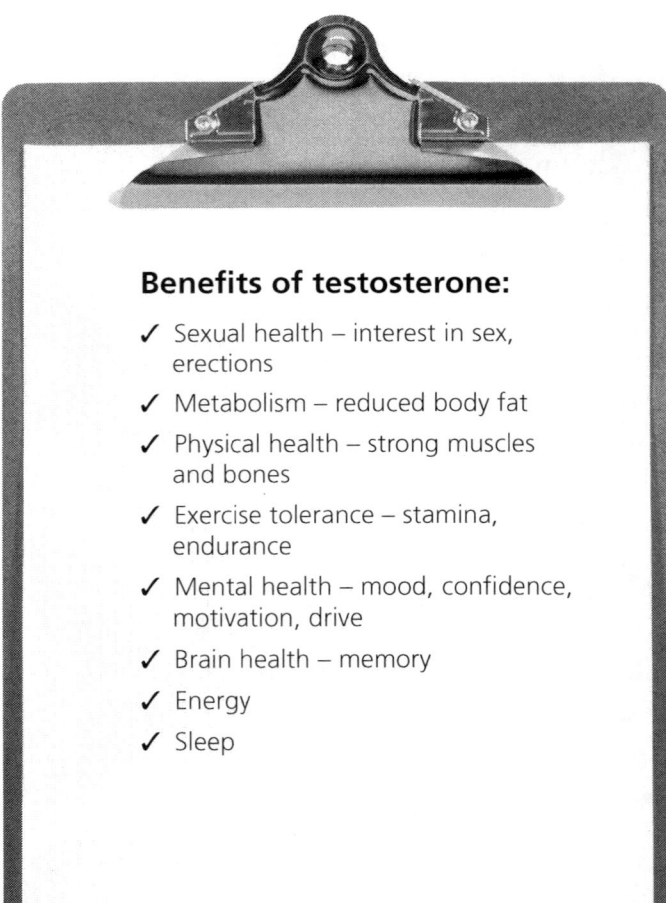

Benefits of testosterone:

- ✓ Sexual health – interest in sex, erections
- ✓ Metabolism – reduced body fat
- ✓ Physical health – strong muscles and bones
- ✓ Exercise tolerance – stamina, endurance
- ✓ Mental health – mood, confidence, motivation, drive
- ✓ Brain health – memory
- ✓ Energy
- ✓ Sleep

men with low testosterone (7). Men with early signs of dementia were given testosterone in an attempt to slow the rate of decline (since we don't have any treatments to actually reverse dementia). What they were surprised to find is that their memory actually improved within 28 days of starting on testosterone. So, if you aren't looking forward to dementia in your future, maintaining optimal testosterone may be helpful (8).

Mental health

Testosterone gives you your confidence, assertiveness, motivation, and competitive drive. One of the early signs when testosterone starts to dip is loss of motivation and confidence. Instead of feeling like taking on the world, you go through the motions and do what you need to do to take care of your family. Inside you feel flat, struggle with self-doubt, second guess your decisions, feel anxious and not quite like yourself.

There is a lot of research to support that lack of testosterone is associated with anxiety and depression. In fact, if you're feeling anxious or depressed, please request a testosterone level before you start antidepressants or anxiety pills to make sure you are treating the right problem!

Physical health

Testosterone is a "build and repair" hormone, and it helps to maintain strong muscles and bones. As testosterone levels drop, strength, stamina, and endurance can be reduced. It can be harder to maintain or build muscle mass. You may find that even if you are working out regularly you aren't able to make gains in the gym the way you had in the past. You may have more post-exercise soreness, take longer to recover after exercise, and be more prone to injuries (that may take longer to heal). Often we chalk these changes up to "getting older", but the real problem may be declining testosterone.

Metabolism

As testosterone levels drop, muscle mass tends to diminish and body fat accumulates. Low testosterone can cause blood sugar problems and predisposes you to diabetes (which makes you gain even more weight).

Sexual health

Testosterone is of course critical to a man's sexual health. Testosterone is important for libido (interest in sex). If your testosterone level is low, you may find that you just don't think about sex very often anymore. Testosterone is also important for erectile function and sexual performance.

Certain health conditions predispose you to having low testosterone, including: obesity, diabetes, high blood pressure, high cholesterol, asthma, sleep apnea, COPD (chronic obstructive pulmonary disease) and prostate disease. Some of these are simply associated with low testosterone and don't actually cause your testosterone to drop, but if you have any of these problems, you and your doctor should be thinking about your testosterone level.

Why Testosterone is Important for Men

How does it feel to have low testosterone (or Low T)?

Let's talk about another patient (we'll call him Stan). Stan is a 53-year-old bank executive. He's still able to keep up at work, but he feels like he's forcing himself to go through the motions and he's just not thriving like he has in the past. He's very health conscious, and he and his wife try to eat well and avoid junk food. He exercises regularly, but he has to force himself to go to the gym (when he used to love it) and he's having more post exercise soreness. He seems to be more prone to injury, and takes longer to recover. He's always been a very high energy guy, but his energy just isn't the same anymore. His sex drive isn't the same either, and while he doesn't have serious problems with erectile function, he has started taking Viagra to help.

When we checked his testosterone level, it was low. He also had elevated inflammation markers, and his blood sugar was creeping up—despite his excellent lifestyle habits.

Once we got his testosterone level restored and his inflammation down, his blood sugar normalized and his energy and sex drive both improved.

Approximately 30% of men over 45 have low testosterone like Stan.

Common symptoms of low T include:

- Fatigue
- Lack of motivation
- Loss of competitive drive

Why Can't I Keep Up Anymore?

Symptoms of low Testosterone:

- ✓ Anxiety
- ✓ Depression
- ✓ Low self-esteem
- ✓ Self-doubt
- ✓ Weight gain
- ✓ Poor memory
- ✓ Trouble with concentration/focus
- ✓ Fatigue
- ✓ Insomnia
- ✓ Loss of motivation/competitive drive
- ✓ Brain fog
- ✓ Feeling older than your age
- ✓ Loss of interest in things you used to enjoy
- ✓ Loss of interest in sex
- ✓ Erectile dysfunction
- ✓ Longer post exercise recovery/soreness
- ✓ More prone to injury
- ✓ Loss of muscle mass
- ✓ Decreased strength
- ✓ Decreased endurance/stamina

Why Testosterone is Important for Men

- Depression
- Anxiety
- Brain Fog
- Lack of focus/concentration
- Weight gain
- Insomnia
- Poor memory
- Loss of interest in sex
- Erectile dysfunction
- Loss of muscle mass
- Decreased strength
- Decreased exercise endurance and stamina
- Feeling "older" than your age
- Loss of interest in things you used to enjoy

Low testosterone is more than just about how you feel—there are some significant health risks associated with low T.

Low T can contribute to:

- Diabetes
- Obesity
- Osteoporosis and hip fractures
- Depression
- Anxiety
- Dementia
- Heart disease
- High cholesterol

Why Can't I Keep Up Anymore?

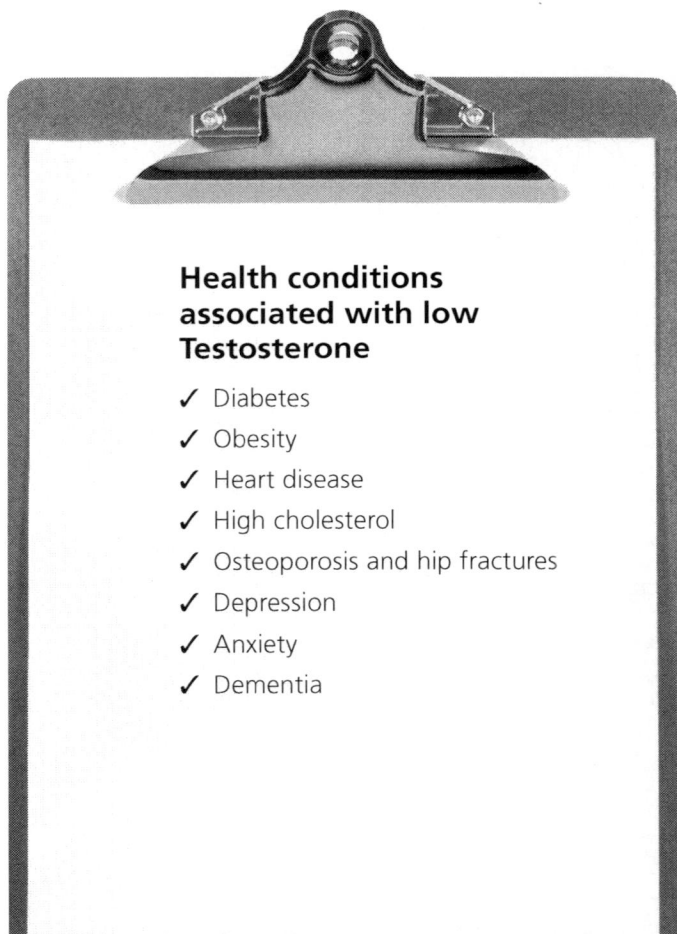

Health conditions associated with low Testosterone

- ✓ Diabetes
- ✓ Obesity
- ✓ Heart disease
- ✓ High cholesterol
- ✓ Osteoporosis and hip fractures
- ✓ Depression
- ✓ Anxiety
- ✓ Dementia

Why Testosterone is Important for Men

There appears to be a fairly strong connection between low T and metabolic syndrome.

Metabolic syndrome is the combination of obesity, high blood sugar, high triglycerides, and high blood pressure. It's associated with an increased risk of heart disease, diabetes and stroke. Men with metabolic syndrome are more likely to have low T, and men with low T are more likely to have metabolic syndrome.(9) We aren't quite sure which is the chicken and which is the egg, but they go together. There are many studies that show that replacing testosterone can improve metabolic syndrome and result in lowered risk of disease.

In his book Super Human, Dave Asprey, the Founder and CEO of Bulletproof (and the guy who coined the term "biohacker") sums it up this way: "You can accept your fate and start sliding downhill at around the age of forty, or you can work to keep your hormones at the levels of someone at his or her peak so you can keep kicking ass long term."

CHAPTER 3

How Does Testosterone Work

You may be surprised to learn that testosterone is made out of cholesterol. Cholesterol is an important building block in your body, although you've been told it is a horrible, artery clogging enemy you should fear. Too much cholesterol may not be a good thing, but very low levels can actually rob you of the ability to produce testosterone! Of course, producing testosterone is not just about having the right ingredients.

All of your hormones, including testosterone, are regulated by a network of checks and balances to make sure that your body is running like a finely tuned, high performance, sports car. Here's how things are supposed to work…

Why Can't I Keep Up Anymore?

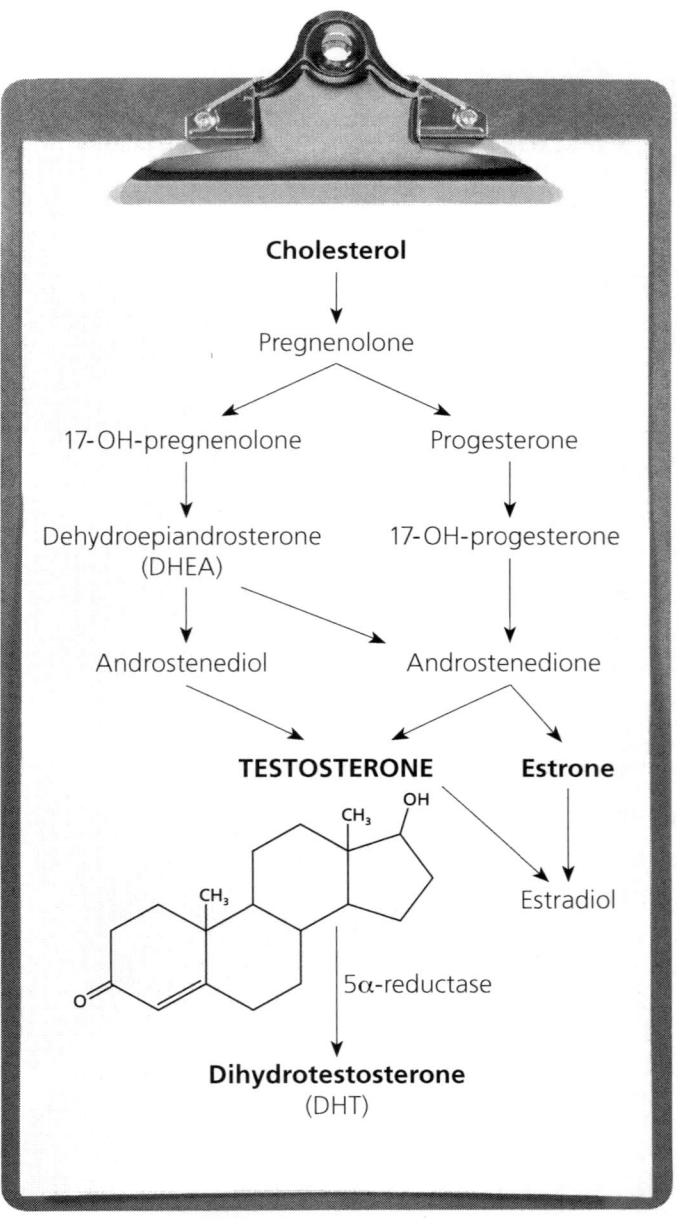

How Does Testosterone Work?

LH

Luteinizing Hormone (LH) comes from the pituitary gland in your brain and travels through the bloodstream to your testes to stimulate more testosterone production. When your brain senses there is enough testosterone in your system, it turns off production. The pituitary gland acts sort of like the thermostat in your home—turning off and on the heat (or in this case, testosterone) to keep the temperature stable.

Sex Hormone Binding Globulin (SHBG)

Testosterone is carried through the bloodstream by a protein called "sex hormone binding globulin" or SHBG. When testosterone is attached to SHBG it becomes inactivated. The testosterone that is floating in your bloodstream without being attached to SHBG is called your "free testosterone," and this is the stuff that activates your cells.

Think of SHBG like a bus—almost all your testosterone is loaded onto the bus, and only a few molecules are left to walk. When testosterone is on the bus, it is not available to activate your cells. Only the testosterone that is walking (the "free" testosterone) can do the job.

If you have a lot of SHBG (a lot of buses), more testosterone will be riding the bus (inactivated) and you'll have less of the free testosterone your cells need, so you won't feel as good. Your total testosterone level is an important number to measure, but we also want to know your free testosterone level.

Estrogen

Testosterone is converted into estrogen by an enzyme called aromatase. If the aromatase enzyme is very active, then more testosterone will be changed into estrogen, leaving you with less testosterone. As you can imagine, having higher estrogen and lower testosterone isn't ideal if you're a man.

Things that increase conversion of testosterone into estrogen:

- Being overweight (especially if you have a lot of weight on your belly)
- Being a diabetic or pre-diabetic
- Drinking alcohol
- Inflammation in your body (from any cause)
- Age
- Poor quality nutrition
- High stress levels
- Lack of exercise

Too much estrogen can cause:

- Fluid retention
- Anxiety
- Irritability
- Feeling more emotional
- Prostate growth
- Erectile dysfunction

How Does Testosterone Work?

- Weight gain (especially in areas where women usually gain weight, like the hips and butt)

Estrogen levels are often low when testosterone is low, and insufficient amounts of estrogen have been associated with bone loss and heart disease.

So once again, having just the right amount is important.

Dihydrotestosterone (DHT)

Testosterone can also be converted into a hormone called DHT by a converting enzyme called 5-alpha reductase.

DHT is actually three times stronger than testosterone and helps with sexual health, energy, and mood, so you won't likely feel bad if your DHT is high. But it's also the hormone associated with male pattern baldness and with prostate growth. If your prostate grows too much, you can have problems emptying your bladder and will find yourself in the Urologist's office.

If your testosterone level is low, then your DHT level is also likely low. If the converting enzyme is overactive, then you may end up converting too much testosterone and end up with high DHT.

Just like the other hormones, too much and not enough are both bad.

DHEA

DHEA is a precursor hormone that can be converted into testosterone. It is an "anti-aging" hormone, and your DHEA level naturally declines with age. This is one of the factors that contribute to a decreased testosterone level as you get older.

Since DHEA is made in your adrenal gland (which makes your other stress hormones, like cortisol and adrenaline), stress can cause DHEA levels to decrease much faster.

In addition, you need adequate levels of DHEA to have optimal growth hormone production.

Human Growth Hormone

Human Growth Hormone (HGH) is very important for healthy aging—it helps maintain a healthy weight and blood sugar metabolism, optimizes sleep, and generally helps slow down the aging process. Unfortunately, this has been used as a drug of abuse by professional athletes and others, and therefore has become difficult for doctors to prescribe. Some doctors have actually been prosecuted for prescribing HGH in patients whose lab values were not severely decreased.

The goal is for you to maintain healthy HGH levels as you age, preferably without the need for a prescription.

CHAPTER 4
What Causes Low T?

There are many reasons that a man may experience a drop in testosterone production.

Age

Testosterone levels peak in early adulthood. After age 30 you can expect your testosterone level to gradually decrease by about 1% every year. If you are 80 years old, it would not be surprising if your testosterone level was low. But if you are in your fifties or below, let's not assume it is due to age! There are a lot of other factors that can cause low testosterone.

Stress

When you are stressed, your body releases cortisol (your main stress hormone) to help you cope.

When we talk about "stress" we include:

Why Can't I Keep Up Anymore?

- Marital stress
- A demanding job
- Being over-scheduled
- Worrying about your kids

These are obvious emotional stresses that you know about. But those aren't the only things that count as stressors in your life. Here are some other things to think about:

- Physical stresses like back pain, injuries and surgeries
- Physiological stress like insomnia, hormone deficiencies, allergies, infections
- Chemical stresses like alcohol, pesticide residues and other toxins that you are exposed to on a regular basis (some that you may not even be aware of)
- Exercise is a good stress, but over-exercising is definitely stressful on your body

All of this stress results in your cortisol level going up to help you cope. In the short term that's a helpful response, but when the stress is day in and day out, cortisol levels can become chronically elevated.

Imagine you are having a fire in the backyard. If you put the right amount of wood on the fire, it's just right. You can sit around it enjoying its warmth, roast marshmallows, whatever you like. But if you put too much wood on there, or gasoline, or if it is exposed to high winds, a pleasant evening

What Causes Low T?

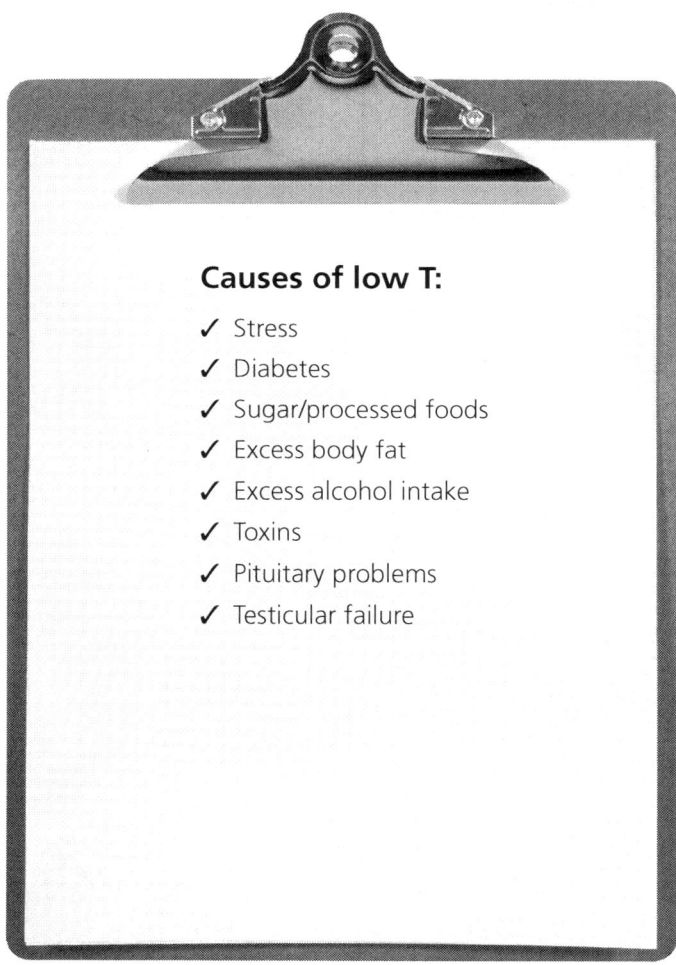

Causes of low T:
- ✓ Stress
- ✓ Diabetes
- ✓ Sugar/processed foods
- ✓ Excess body fat
- ✓ Excess alcohol intake
- ✓ Toxins
- ✓ Pituitary problems
- ✓ Testicular failure

around the fire can quickly shift to a dangerous inferno damaging everything it comes into contact with.

High cortisol shuts down testosterone production (after all, in your body's infinite wisdom, if there is a highly stressful time like a famine, this is not the time to be procreating!)

Testosterone is a 'build and repair' hormone that helps keep you young. Cortisol is a 'wear and tear' hormone that speeds up the aging process. They are opposites and need to be in balance.

Excessive alcohol intake

Alcohol is poison to your testicles. In excess, alcohol can reduce testosterone production, impair fertility and even cause cell damage in the testes.(1) Excess alcohol increases the conversion of testosterone into estrogen. Limit your alcohol intake to no more than 2 drinks a day.

Sugar/processed foods

Sugar is a toxin. There are many reasons that you should limit the sugar in your diet. Testosterone production is one of them.

When you eat a diet full of sugar and processed foods, you are typically not providing your body with the nutrients it needs for your cells to do their jobs (including producing testosterone). And a diet high in sugar and processed foods is also a recipe to develop problems with blood sugar, which can reduce testosterone production.

What Causes Low T?

The good news is that healthy eating can help turn this around!

Excess body fat

When you gain fat, especially around your belly, we used to think it was just extra weight for you to carry around. Now we understand that those fat cells are very metabolically active, kind of like little factories pumping out inflammatory chemicals into your bloodstream.

These inflammatory chemicals interfere with insulin function, so you develop more blood sugar problems, which makes you gain more weight (especially around your belly).

That spare tire you are carrying around is also an estrogen producing factory! (2) Your belly fat is taking your testosterone and converting it into estrogen. If you are growing 'man boobs' then you can make this diagnosis without a blood test!

Losing weight will do more than affect your belt size; it will also help you to transform your hormone pattern.

Illicit drugs

If you needed another reason to clean up your act, here you go. Most illicit drugs have a negative effect on testosterone. Methamphetamines, including "meth" and MDMA (or ecstasy), lower testosterone levels. Cocaine and other opioids (including prescription pain medications) are well known to lower testosterone levels. Illegal anabolic steroids that you get from the guy at the gym—ditto. Take enough of those and the drop in testosterone could be permanent.

Marijuana

There is mixed news on marijuana. Some studies show a dramatic reduction in testosterone, but some studies found no problem. There is evidence that sperm count and fertility are reduced in marijuana users, and there also seems to an increase in estrogen levels. 'Gynecomastia' is the medical term for man boobs. If you have this problem, you may want to rethink your use of weed.

Lack of sexual activity

While low testosterone can cause you to lose desire for sex, it seems that lack of sexual activity may cause lower testosterone! (3) During sex and masturbation, testosterone levels increase and then go back down to normal after ejaculation. In one study, abstaining from sexual activity (with or without a partner) for 3 months caused a reduction in testosterone level, but the level improved again when sexual activity resumed.

Diabetes

Men who have diabetes have an increased risk of low testosterone. And men with low testosterone have an increased risk for developing diabetes. (4) This is because insulin (the hormone that regulates your blood sugar) and testosterone affect each other.

If your testosterone level is not optimal, it's quite possible that you'll find your blood sugar level is starting to creep up too, and sometimes it's hard to know which is the chicken and the egg—is the blood sugar problem causing the dip in testosterone or vice versa. Either way, optimizing blood sugar metabolism can help to improve testosterone function.

Sleep apnea

Since testosterone is mainly released at night while you are sleeping, if you are not getting into a nice deep sleep state, you may not be properly releasing testosterone. You may have no idea that you are waking up many times during the night! Talk to your doctor about getting a sleep study if you think you could have this problem, especially if your bed partner tells you that you snore. Not everyone with sleep apnea snores, but snoring is an important clue.

Medications

Narcotic pain medications (including morphine, codeine, hydrocodone or oxycodone) suppress testosterone production by shutting down the message from your brain telling your body to make testosterone. Low testosterone often results in a lowered pain threshold, more inflammation and slower healing. Unfortunately, this may result in increasing doses of pain medication, and getting caught in a cycle that can be hard to resolve.

Cholesterol-lowering medications such as atorvastatin, simvastatin and other "statin" drugs may also lower testosterone levels. Cholesterol is an important ingredient for testosterone production, so when cholesterol is too low, testosterone production is impaired. If your total cholesterol level is below 130mg/dl, it could be a problem for your hormones.

Certain medications for Attention Deficit Disorder (ADD) and some anti-depressants may also cause problems with testosterone. Talk with your doctor if you are concerned that this may be the case for you.

Environmental toxins

Every day we are all exposed to tens of thousands of manmade chemicals that were never found on planet earth before WWII. Many of these chemicals are "endocrine disruptors," meaning they can screw up your hormones.

We know that many of these contribute to low testosterone in men (5), but it is very hard to prove scientifically. It's not like we can take a whole bunch of men, douse them in chemicals and then measure their testosterone levels to see what happens! We do know from animal studies that lower testosterone levels, lower sperm count, and lower fertility results from exposure to many of these chemicals.

For example, triclosan is the ingredient found in anti-bacterial soap, which was really popular a few years ago. Have

What Causes Low T?

you noticed that it is no longer available? Go to the store and look for "anti-bacterial" soap. It is gone. Triclosan was quietly removed from the market because we had enough proof that it was contributing to hormone problems, and specifically reducing testosterone levels.(6)

Another hormone-disrupting chemical is Atrazine. This is an herbicide, commonly sprayed on crops. Atrazine runs off into streams causing feminization and reduction of testosterone in a wide range of animals, including mammals. It can actually turn boy frogs into girl frogs. (7)

But what exactly does Atrazine do to boy humans? We don't really know, because how would we do the study? Would you be willing to sign up to be exposed to varying amounts to see how it affects your manhood???

And there are THOUSANDS more chemicals that could be affecting our hormones. Unfortunately, the chemical companies don't have to prove that their chemical is safe for humans, because most of the time we aren't supposed to be consuming it. For example, atrazine isn't supposed to be eaten, but it gets in our water and into our bodies anyway.

The burden is on the consumer to PROVE that they have been harmed by a particular product or chemical. The big problem is that you are exposed to thousands of chemicals every day in various combinations. How could you ever prove that your medical issue (low testosterone, cancer, etc.) is caused by that company's chemical?

Unless there are a whole bunch of people with similar

health issues in a small area it can be impossible. Even if there are people with similar issues in a small area it is still very hard to prove (remember Erin Brokovitch?).

Flushing chemicals from your system and avoiding exposure when possible are important, but not guaranteed to completely resolve the hormone imbalances that have taken years to develop.

Pituitary problems

Your pituitary gland is the part of your brain responsible for sending out hormone signals to the rest of the body. It makes LH which goes to the testes to tell them to make more testosterone. If your pituitary isn't functioning properly, it may not be making LH, so your body COULD make testosterone, but your cells are just not being told to make it.

In men, high levels of stress can suppress pituitary function. Once the stress resolves, the system can get back to normal and testosterone production can improve. This is not uncommon.

Less commonly, there can be damage to the pituitary gland. For example, if you have had head trauma, like a concussion, the pituitary is susceptible to injury. It is situated at the bottom of the brain flush up against your skull, so it can be bashed against the bone of your skull and may not work properly after. This is something seen in football players who have repeated head blows over their career.

Rarely, tumors can form in the pituitary gland. The most common is called a pituitary adenoma, which is a benign

What Causes Low T?

tumor (not cancerous) and is typically slow growing. The problem is that it's deep in your brain in a tiny important area that doesn't lend itself well to surgical removal. Most often we follow it along and manage the hormone problems that it causes.

A pituitary adenoma can be evaluated by looking at your prolactin level. Prolactin is a hormone made in the pituitary gland. A very elevated prolactin level is a clue to a possible pituitary tumor, and typically a brain MRI will be done to help with the diagnosis.

To determine whether a pituitary problem exists, an LH level can be done. It is important to do this test before testosterone therapy is started. Taking testosterone replacement turns off the pituitary messaging system and causes the LH level to go down (which isn't necessarily a problem, it just means we lose the ability to judge your natural LH production).

Primary testicular failure

Another problem is that your testes may stop working. We call this primary testicular failure, or primary hypogonadism. (If your testes work fine but your brain isn't sending the message we call it secondary hypogonadism).

We can tell the difference by measuring your LH level. If your LH level is high and your testosterone level is low, it means that your brain is yelling at your testes but they simply aren't responding. One reason for testicular failure, which may be more common than we realize, is an autoimmune problem, which means that your immune system is inappropriately attacking the cells in your testes. We don't have readily available tests for these antibodies (although some specialty labs are developing these tests) so we can't always make this diagnosis with certainty.

As you can see, there are a lot of different factors that can contribute to low T. If all we do is measure your testosterone level and prescribe testosterone replacement, we aren't really getting at the underlying factors that caused the problem in the first place. We can't always restore testosterone levels naturally, but if we don't address the factors that caused the problem we'll never get the best results!

This is a really common problem that I see. You may have had your testosterone level tested (if you were lucky) and been told it is low. You may have been prescribed testosterone gel and you may feel somewhat better but still not great, because your body is still too inflamed, or full of toxins, or whatever the underlying issues are. We can't always correct testosterone levels naturally, but it seems important to me to try!

It's possible you were tested and told that your testosterone level is normal (although you can see that you are sitting right down at the bottom end of normal). You don't need a medical degree to imagine that you could probably feel better if your testosterone was a little higher up in the normal range! But typically you'll just be told you're normal, and no further recommendations will be given. You're just left to live your life with less vitality, oomph, and vigor, less

What Causes Low T?

sexual function and increased risk of chronic disease. How frustrating! Fortunately, now you know there is another way.

Let's talk more in the next chapter about how to get the right diagnosis.

CHAPTER 5

How to Diagnose Low T

Labs to evaluate/follow treatment

If you aren't feeling your best and want your testosterone level to be evaluated, blood work can give you the answer. But it takes more than just a testosterone level to get the full picture. If you doctor wants to measure just your testosterone and then prescribe testosterone replacement, you aren't really getting optimal treatment.

These are the labs that I recommend:

Total testosterone—the total amount of testosterone in your bloodstream. The "normal" range is actually very controversial. In fact, over the 13 years that I have been doing testosterone replacement, the "normal" level with LabCorp went from 200-800 to 350-1197, then in the past year went back to 300-800. You can see that even the lab can't decide what is normal!

The most commonly accepted "normal" range is 300-1000ng/dl. (1)

Why Can't I Keep Up Anymore?

A study of healthy men ages 19-40 found the average testosterone level was 748 ng/dl. The bottom 2.5 percentile level was 348, and anything below this was considered low. (2) That means 97.5% of men between19-40 have a higher testosterone level than 348. If your testosterone level was 349, would you be happy with that definition of normal?

In this study, men with low testosterone levels had higher rates of sexual dysfunction, difficulty climbing stairs, slow walking speed, frailty, and diabetes than those with normal levels. Remember these were not elderly men—they were all under 40!

Another thing to keep in mind is that some labs change the "normal" range depending on your age. I recommend staying in the normal range for a 40-year-old no matter your age.

Most doctors who are working to balance your hormones have a goal of testosterone in the upper half of the normal range.

Knowing your total testosterone is not nearly enough information to decide whether you are 'optimal' or how to go about making things optimal.

Free testosterone—most of your testosterone (about 97%) is carried around your bloodstream by a protein called SHBG. In a previous chapter we talked about how SHBG is like a bus—only the testosterone that is walking (the "free" testosterone) can do the job.

We can measure your free testosterone level, and this is actually more important that the total amount!

You may have a lot of total testosterone, but if it is mostly bound to SHBG, you won't have much of the free testosterone that your body needs.

Here is another way to think about it. Let's say you have a lot of wealth (testosterone) but all your money is tied up in real estate. You have no liquidity. You don't have available cash (free testosterone) to spend freely when you need it. You won't feel good.

On the other hand, your total testosterone may be low normal, but if you don't have much SHBG, you'll still have enough free testosterone to do the job. This is like only having $1000 to your name, but it is all cash in your pocket, so it's immediately available if you need it. You may feel just fine.

Since free testosterone is the one that activates your cells, your free testosterone level is more closely correlated with your symptoms than the total testosterone.

SHBG (sex hormone binding globulin)—we can measure your SHBG level to see how many "buses" you have in your fleet, which helps us understand the free testosterone result.

Let's say, for example, that your total testosterone is 600 (not bad) but your SHBG is very high—this will result in a free testosterone level that is low normal, and you probably won't feel great despite the normal testosterone level.

Estrogen—You actually have several different kinds of estrogen in your body. Estradiol is the strongest estrogen and is the one that is most typically measured.

Why Can't I Keep Up Anymore?

The "normal" level of estrogen is also controversial. Different labs will have very different "normal" ranges, and this has been very perplexing for doctors and patients.

Men need some estrogen (it helps protect your bones, just as it does for women) but not too much or you can have fluid retention, breast growth, and irritability. According to the medical literature, estradiol below 20pg/ml and above 30pg/ml was associated with more risks, so I typically look for an estrogen level in the 20s. (3)

Estrogen is made from testosterone, so when testosterone is low, estrogen is typically low. As testosterone levels improve, estrogen levels will also go up; but it's important to make sure they don't go up too high!

If we give you more testosterone and your body flips it into estrogen, your testosterone level won't go up as much as you would expect. Instead, your estrogen will get higher! The higher estrogen works against the testosterone (and contributes to erectile dysfunction)(4) so you won't get the results that you are hoping for.

This happens all the time in doctor's offices, and may have already happened to you. Your total testosterone level is low and estrogen is never measured. Testosterone gel is prescribed, but you don't really feel better, and your doctor doesn't really have anything more to add (other than trying an increased dose—but now you can predict what will happen…More estrogen!)

There are a few things that make it more likely you'll flip your testosterone to estrogen, including having belly fat, being a diabetic (or prediabetic), inflammation in your body, or just genetics.

Addressing these issues can help, and there are some supplements and medications that can slow the conversion of testosterone to estrogen. In some men who have low testosterone because of too much estrogen conversion, slowing down the conversion may be the only treatment required to get you back into balance (you may not need testosterone replacement!)

I believe that monitoring estrogen is a crucial part of addressing testosterone issues. But unfortunately, it is usually not measured. You will need to specifically request that an estradiol level be tested.

LH (Luteinizing Hormone)—remember from earlier, this is the hormone from your pituitary gland that tells your testes to make testosterone. It is important to measure this hormone BEFORE you start on testosterone replacement, because once you are on it your LH will become suppressed by the treatment and will be low.

The initial level (before treatment) helps us understand WHY your testosterone is low.

A high level means your testes aren't working properly, and your brain is "yelling" to get more testosterone.

A low level means your pituitary gland is not sending the right message. This is an important distinction to make and can affect your treatment options. Unfortunately, it is not typically measured in most doctors' offices, so you will need to request it.

Why Can't I Keep Up Anymore?

DHT (Dihydrotestosterone)—is made out of testosterone. It is three times as strong as testosterone and gives much of the benefits that we are looking for from testosterone—sexual health, energy, and mood for example. If testosterone is low, DHT is typically low and as the testosterone level is normalized, the DHT should improve also.

If you have an enlarged prostate, you need to be aware that several of the medicines that are used for benign prostate hypertrophic (BPH) block the conversion of testosterone to DHT, which can help shrink the size of your prostate.

Pills for hair loss also work this way, because DHT is the hormone that triggers hair loss in men who are genetically predisposed.

If you are on any of these medications including finasteride (trade name Propecia) and dutasteride (trade name Avodart), your DHT level will be low regardless of your testosterone level, and it won't go up even if your testosterone level is boosted.

The most common side effect of these medicines includes impotence, decreased libido, and decreased volume of ejaculation. If these are some of your symptoms, it could be from the medicine and not from low T.

Here's the compromise: using a low dose of finasteride or related medications can shrink your prostate so you can pee (somewhat important!) and can also help to reduce hair loss (also very important to many men).

If you feel okay, I suggest taking the lowest dose that seems to do the trick while optimizing your testosterone level. But be aware that your DHT level will be low, so no point in monitoring it.

This hormone level is not typically measured in most doctors' offices, so you will likely have to specifically ask for it.

DHEA (Dihydroepiandrosterone)—this is an 'anti-aging' hormone made in your adrenal glands, and it naturally declines with age and with stress. On the lab results, the "normal" range is adjusted based on your age.

If you are 25 years old, the "normal" range is approximately 100-450 mcg/dL (each lab has a slightly different range) and if you are 75 years old, the "normal" range may be 30-150 mcg/dL.

I recommend trying to keep your DHEA level in the optimal range for a 40-year-old, approximately 150-250 mcg/dL, no matter your age. This is another one you'll have to ask to have tested.

CBC (complete blood count)—your blood count measures your red blood cells, white blood cells, and platelet count.

Testosterone stimulates your bone marrow to make more red blood cells, and this makes your blood "thicker" (typically we like a little bit of blood "thinning", which is what a baby aspirin does for example).

We look at your hematocrit (hct) and hemoglobin (hgb) levels to understand how many red blood cells are in your blood, and what the "thickness" is.

If you already have a higher hemoglobin level before we

start treatment and then the level goes up even more, your blood can "thicken" too much and we worry about you getting a blood clot. This is controversial, and we're still trying to figure out exactly how much of a problem this may be.

While the research is being done to answer the question (which could take years) I typically don't allow my patients to walk around with a really high blood count just in case. No one wants to have stroke, and we have a pretty simple solution—donate blood. Regular blood donation is good for the community and good for you.

Some men are not good candidates for blood donation— for example if you've recently visited a foreign country they may not take your blood. There is a way around this, however. You can get a prescription for a therapeutic phlebotomy (phlebotomy is just the medical word for a blood draw). They'll take your blood but then throw it out. A nuisance, but better than a stroke......

CBC levels are routinely done in all doctors' offices and should be no problem to get, but it is best to ask just to make sure it gets done.

PSA (prostate specific antigen)—a blood test to screen for prostate cancer.

Honestly, it isn't a great test. Most of the time if your PSA is up it just means that there is inflammation in your prostate, which can be from things like having sex last night, going on a long bike ride, or having a low grade infection in the area. It is probably NOT due to prostate cancer. But, it is the only blood test we have available, and if it is elevated then at least we have some indication that further evaluation should be done.

The next step, if you have a high PSA level, is another blood test for the '% free PSA'—the value here can help predict whether or not cancer is likely. A digital rectal exam (the dreaded rubber glove exam) to feel your prostate is also important.

Testosterone replacement doesn't increase the risk of getting prostate cancer, but if you have prostate cancer right now, starting testosterone replacement is not the best idea. Doctors are obligated to do some sort of evaluation for prostate cancer before starting on testosterone replacement, especially in older men.

More advanced labs

There is a wide range of more advanced lab testing available to understand about the underlying factors that led you to having low T. Vitamin and mineral deficiencies, such as low zinc, can cause low T. Blood sugar markers, inflammatory markers, and cortisol levels can give clues (more about cortisol in chapter 9). There are tests to look at levels of toxins in your body and to evaluate how well your liver detox pathways clear toxins. These are not tests that you will be able to get from your regular doctor. You'll need to find a Functional Medicine doctor for this kind of in depth approach to your health.

Why Can't I Keep Up Anymore?

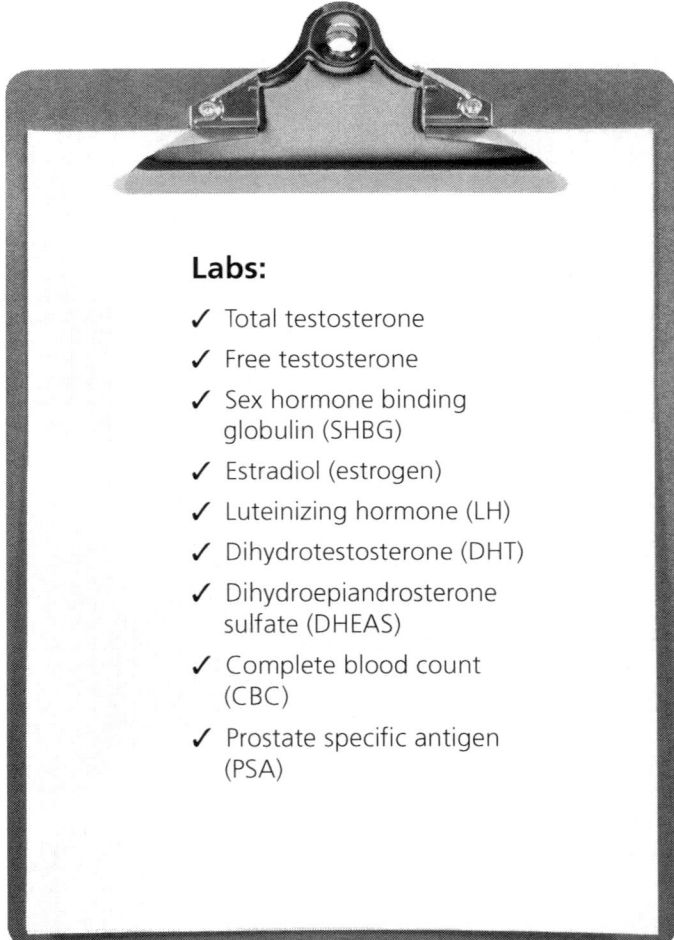

Labs:

- ✓ Total testosterone
- ✓ Free testosterone
- ✓ Sex hormone binding globulin (SHBG)
- ✓ Estradiol (estrogen)
- ✓ Luteinizing hormone (LH)
- ✓ Dihydrotestosterone (DHT)
- ✓ Dihydroepiandrosterone sulfate (DHEAS)
- ✓ Complete blood count (CBC)
- ✓ Prostate specific antigen (PSA)

CHAPTER 6

Medical Treatment For Low T

Let's talk about another patient (we'll call him Michael). Michael is a 40-year-old divorce attorney. He has been gaining weight, but he really doesn't have the motivation to exercise. He feels tired most of the time, and his sex drive is markedly decreased. Erections are less strong, although he can still perform with the help of Viagra. He feels anxious (which is new) and has lost interest in some of the activities he used to enjoy, like playing basketball with his friends at the Y.

He went to his doctor, who listened to his complaints and diagnosed him with depression. The antidepressant his doctor prescribed isn't making him feel better. In fact, the medication makes him feel kind of like a "zombie" and killed the rest his sex drive.

When he came to see me, I found that Michael had a testosterone level of 250, which is very low for a 40-year-old. His free testosterone and estrogen were also low. His LH was high, indicating that his testes are not able to make testosterone, so he was started on testosterone replacement.

Within the first couple of weeks, he felt his energy improve, his mood got better, and he was able to focus at work and handle stress better. Within a few months, he lost 10 pounds and came off the anti-depressant.

When men have low testosterone, there are actually a number of treatment options besides just testosterone replacement.

One option (especially if your testosterone level is low normal, but not extremely low) is to work on your lifestyle habits and add some targeted nutritional supplements (based on your labs results) and give this a couple of months to see if you feel better and your testosterone level starts to improve.

If this is unsuccessful, then there are a number of medical options.

- Clomiphene—a prescription pill to boost testosterone production
- Human Chorionic Gonadotrophin (HCG)—injections to boost testosterone production
- Topical testosterone gel, cream or patches
- Testosterone injections
- Testosterone pellets

1. Clomiphene

This is a prescription drug (brand name "Clomid") that is more commonly used to treat fertility problems in women, because it stimulates ovulation.

Medical Treatment for Low T

In men, it's also used for fertility problems, because it stimulates the pituitary gland to make LH (luteinizing hormone), which tells your testes to make more testosterone and boost sperm count. If you already have a high LH level, then your body is already trying to do this for you naturally, so this treatment is not likely going to work for you.

If your LH is low normal, then this is something that you can try. Your blood work should be retested in about three weeks to see if your testosterone level has gone up. You can also measure LH to make sure it has gone up appropriately with the treatment. The dose can be adjusted to optimize the treatment.

It doesn't work for everyone, so if it's not doing the job for you, you can move on to another one of the options. If it's working well, you can continue for around six months (while you are also working on your lifestyle habits!) and then stop to see if you have reset your system and can maintain testosterone naturally. If not, you can restart or move to another one of the options to optimize testosterone levels.

Clomiphene may be a good option for younger men who want to be able to start a family since testosterone replacement can inhibit sperm production and reduce fertility. (1) This is especially an issue if sperm count isn't great in the beginning (likely due to the same issues that caused a young man to have low testosterone in the first place), so if appropriate, clomiphene (or HCG—see below) may be considered first, and testosterone reserved if these are not effective.

Why Can't I Keep Up Anymore?

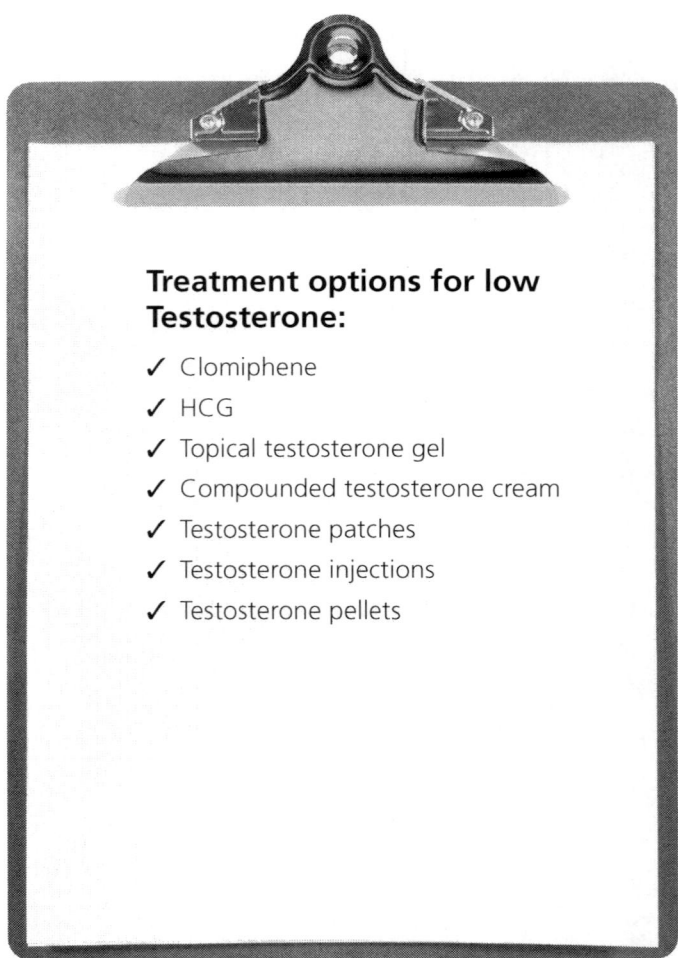

Treatment options for low Testosterone:

- ✓ Clomiphene
- ✓ HCG
- ✓ Topical testosterone gel
- ✓ Compounded testosterone cream
- ✓ Testosterone patches
- ✓ Testosterone injections
- ✓ Testosterone pellets

Medical Treatment for Low T

Please note that being on testosterone is NOT birth control and while sperm count may be decreased it is not turned off!

This is a newer treatment and we don't have research to show the effects of taking clomiphene for the long term. We know the effects of low T, so raising your testosterone level is desirable, but we don't know if long term use of clomiphene has some unforeseen effects. It is not something that is used commonly, so your doctor may not be familiar with this option.

Pros

- A pill (no injections)
- Naturally increases your own testosterone production
- May help "reset" your system to help you naturally produce testosterone on your own
- No negative effect on fertility

Cons

- Doesn't work for everyone
- No long term studies

2. HCG (Human Chorionic Gonadotropin)

HCG stimulates your own testosterone production by telling the testes to make more testosterone. It isn't a good choice if your LH level is already high, because your body is already trying to do this, but if your LH level is low normal, this can be tried. Your testosterone level should be rechecked in about three weeks to see if it's working, and the dose can be adjusted for best results.

HCG is given by subcutaneous injections at home, 2-3 times weekly.

This is another good option for younger men who want to be able to start a family. The HCG is not just stimulating the testes to make more testosterone, but it also stimulates sperm production (and is used as a fertility treatment for men with low sperm count).

Pros

- No negative effect on fertility (and may actually help boost sperm count)
- Naturally increases your own testosterone production

Cons

- Doesn't work for everyone
- Requires injections

3. Topical Testosterone

Topical testosterone is readily available, and comes in several different forms:

- Gel pumps
- Gel packets
- Underarm application

Medical Treatment for Low T

- Patches
- Compounded cream

The most common form of topical testosterone is a gel that is applied to areas like shoulders, upper arm, or abdomen once daily. Care is necessary when using topical testosterone because the gel can rub off on women, children, and pets. Since men need a large dose of testosterone, even a fraction of the dose can be significant for women or children. In an effort to minimize this, some gels are applied to the scrotum or underarm area.

Measuring your testosterone level is a little tricky with topical testosterone because your blood levels will be inconsistent. The blood level spikes up after about two hours, and then drops fairly quickly, so your lab result will vary depending on how many hours since you applied the gel, and even where you applied it.

You may not feel the fluctuation, (the testosterone is in your tissues, it just doesn't stay in your bloodstream), so the blood level is not always an accurate measurement of the testosterone in your body. It is important to consider how you are feeling and not just make dosing decisions based on a blood test.

I typically recommend having your blood test done first thing in the morning before applying the testosterone. Since this will represent the "trough" level (the lowest dip in your testosterone before you apply the next dose) we expect your level to be in the lower half of the normal range, but not

Why Can't I Keep Up Anymore?

below normal. You know that your level will be higher again once you apply the next dose.

Estrogen patches work very well in women, but testosterone patches in men aren't the same. In theory, the patch should release a stable amount of testosterone over the course of the day, which is desirable. However, none of the patients I've tried on patches have elected to stay on them—they've all changed to other forms of testosterone with better results. The same is true for the gel intended to be applied to the scrotum or to the underarm area. I am willing to prescribe these if someone wants to try them, but they haven't been popular with my patients.

Topical gels may be covered by your health insurance if your testosterone level is low enough. If you don't have insurance, or if your testosterone level is not low enough to meet your insurance company's threshold, these gel preparations can be very cost prohibitive.

Testosterone is also available from a compounding pharmacy. Compounding pharmacies are specialized pharmacies that make the testosterone gel or cream based on a doctor's prescription. We can make the concentration of testosterone stronger (meaning a higher dose in a smaller amount of gel or cream), and this seems to help with absorption. We can also change the type of cream or gel the testosterone is mixed in if you have developed a reaction.

Compounding pharmacies are controversial. Since each prescription is unique, they can't be FDA approved. Even though the testosterone used to make up the prescription is

FDA approved, the final product is not. I have found that in some cases the topical creams give a better result that the topical gels, but not all doctors are comfortable working with a compounding pharmacy and prefer to stick to the standard formulations. If you're going to use a compounding pharmacy, I recommend looking for one that is PCAB accredited (Pharmacy Compounding Accreditation Board). This voluntary accreditation demonstrates a commitment to meeting the highest industry standards for quality and safety.

Pros

- Readily available
- May be covered by insurance based on your baseline testosterone level

Cons

- Results not as consistent as injections or pellets
- Tricky for your doctor to get an accurate testosterone level
- Could cause elevated testosterone in family members

4. Testosterone injections

This is the most popular choice of testosterone replacement in my office.

Testosterone cypionate is the most commonly used injectable form of testosterone. Testosterone is attached to a molecule called 'cypionate', which holds the testosterone in your body. Your body naturally chops off the cypionate bit by bit over the next week, gradually releasing testosterone into your blood stream.

Injections are given at home, usually once a week. Typically, the level will increase quickly after an injection, and then gradually go down. Some men don't even notice the changes, but some men feel great for a couple of days, and then feel worse for the second half of the week. If this is the case for you, you can split the dose—use half the dose twice weekly (you could even give yourself 1/7th the dose daily, but not many people sign up for that!).

Some doctors will have you come into the office to get the injection, and they give a bigger dose once every two weeks or once a month. This often results in a very high level for the first week, but then the level starts dropping, and a dropping testosterone level doesn't feel good. This is mostly done for convenience (it is inconvenient to have to go into the doctor's office weekly). Doing the injection yourself at home once weekly seems to be the best balance between frequent injections, stable testosterone levels, and good results.

Testosterone cypionate is FDA approved for intramuscular injections, typically given into the gluteus muscle of the buttock or the upper, outer thigh. Many men prefer subcutaneous injections (under the skin of the stomach). While not FDA approved for subcutaneous injections, this is easier and less uncomfortable to administer, and the needle is much smaller. In my clinical experience, these subcutaneous injections work well and result in good testosterone levels without any more problems than we experience with IM injections. Occasionally there can be bruising or soreness at the site of injections, but generally these work well, and we get few complaints.

Testosterone levels are easier to measure in a blood test than the topical gels, but timing is still very important. Typically we measure testosterone levels midweek between injections. We are looking for a level in the upper quartile of the normal range. If blood work is done at the end of the week (before the next injection), the testosterone level may be below the halfway point, but shouldn't drop down too low.

Testosterone by injection is often the least expensive option. The price of a 10ml vial (which will last for several months) ranges from $35-$100 if you are paying out of pocket.

PROS:

- It is a guarantee that your testosterone level will go up with the right dose
- It is easier to measure your testosterone level, although the level still varies over the week
- Most men get good results
- Less expensive

CONS:

- Levels vary over the week
- Requires injections

5. Testosterone pellets

Another option is testosterone pellets. Testosterone is fused into pellets (they look like Tic-Tacs) which are inserted under the skin of the upper buttock in a minor office procedure.

The skin is numbed with lidocaine (this stings for a few seconds) then a tiny incision is made in the upper/outer buttock (just above where your pant pocket sits), and the pellets slide through the incision and under the skin. There is swelling and tenderness for a few days, and there is often a little bruising. You'll be asked to avoid vigorous exercise for 4-5 days after insertion, to help prevent loss of any pellets until this skin seals up (since we don't use stitches).

As blood flows over the pellets, the testosterone is gradually melted out and into your bloodstream at a nice steady pace. In fact, pellets give us the most stable blood level of testosterone.

Another nice thing about pellets is that the rate of testosterone release is varied based on blood flow. For example, if you are exercising, there will be a temporary increase in blood flow, so there will be a temporary increase in the rate of testosterone release. This mimics your body's natural response to exercise.

As the pellets melt away, the testosterone level will start to come down. At a typical dose, the effect of the pellets lasts for 3-5 months (higher doses will last longer).

There can be some complications with pellets. Rarely there can be an infection, which is a risk any time there is a cut in the skin. The symptoms typically are noted 3-5 days after insertion, but fortunately this is uncommon.

Occasionally, the body can react to the pellets as a foreign body and develop inflammation, with redness, swelling, itching, and discomfort. This often resolves on its own, but can be treated with antihistamines or steroids, if necessary. This can sometimes be confused with an infection.

Sometimes the body "rejects" the pellets, and 3-5 weeks after insertion some of the pellets can be extruded out through the skin. Usually this happens if the pellets are placed a little too superficially, and is very uncommon if proper insertion technique is used.

Pellets are a great form of testosterone replacement—a nice stable level that lasts for several months without having to think about it or do anything.

PROS

- Stable testosterone level
- After the insertion, can forget about it for months
- Guaranteed to increase your testosterone level

CONS

- More expensive
- Requires an office procedure
- Some swelling, bruising, and mild discomfort for a couple of days
- Can't be removed if there is a problem
- Risk of infection or inflammatory reaction

Why Can't I Keep Up Anymore?

Will your testosterone replacement be covered by insurance?

Well, it depends on your baseline level. If your testosterone level is below 200 ng/dL, your insurance company will likely pay for your testosterone replacement. If your level is below 300ng/dL, your insurance may cover it. If your level is above 300 ng/dL, it is unlikely that you are going to be able to get the testosterone covered. Fortunately, there are options for testosterone replacement that are not overly expensive, and knowing the range of options is helpful. (It's always nice to have options!)

6. Estrogen blockers

If you are making an adequate amount of testosterone, but converting too much into estrogen, both your estrogen and testosterone levels may be in the "normal" range, but you won't likely feel great. If we just give you testosterone replacement, you'll likely just convert more testosterone into estrogen and not get the results you are looking for. This is why it is so important to know your testosterone level AND your estrogen level.

If this is the case for you, improving lifestyle habits is very important (including losing weight, improving blood sugar metabolism, and reducing inflammation).

If the problem is mild, there is a natural herbal supplement called chrysin that can help reduce estrogen production.

Sometimes prescription medications are required. Anastrazole (brand name Arimidex) or letrozole (brand name Femara) reduce the conversion of testosterone to estrogen, and can allow testosterone levels to go up and estrogen levels to go down—so you may not end up needing testosterone replacement therapy.

Why doesn't testosterone replacement always fix the symptoms?

I commonly see men who come in complaining of not feeling great, but they are already on testosterone, or already tried it in the past and didn't really feel better. Their doctor may have tried to increase or decrease the dose, but didn't really have the answer. And typically, just their testosterone level was checked.

If your doctor is only following your testosterone level (and not your estrogen level), that is a red flag that you are not getting the best care. In fairness to your doctor, following your testosterone level is all they have been trained to do. Even if you asked for an estrogen level to be done, they haven't been trained to evaluate estrogen in men (to know what is optimal) or how to fix it if it is not.

Here are just a few reasons why you may not be getting the results you expect from your testosterone replacement:

- Incorrect dose (especially with topical gel, since it is harder to accurately measure blood levels)
- The testosterone is getting converted into too much estrogen
- SHBG is inactivating your testosterone so you don't feel it (causing a low free testosterone)

Why Can't I Keep Up Anymore?

- Your cortisol level is too high
- Your cortisol level is too low
- The testosterone is making your untreated sleep apnea worse
- You have too much inflammation in your body
- You are deficient in certain vitamins or minerals like B12, B6, or zinc
- Your thyroid level is low
- You have a low grade chronic infection like digestive yeast overgrowth or Lyme disease
- You have heavy metals, like lead or mercury, in your body

You can see that sometimes, simply replacing testosterone without looking at the big picture can overlook some pretty important factors! Fortunately, a Functional Medicine doctor can help you work through these issues. It is not necessary for everyone to be tested for all of these things (we choose the tests based on your symptoms and history). But if you're already on testosterone replacement and still not feeling great, it is good to know that there are other factors that can be addressed to help you get the great results you're looking for!

Side Effects and Risks of T Replacement

Testosterone replacement is generally well tolerated. Finding the best dose and best route of administration can take a little bit of trial and error, but most men feel significantly better—often in ways that are hard to measure: more energy, mood, vitality, motivation, sexual interest and performance....

With anything in medicine, however, there are risks and benefits.

Here are some of the potential problems with testosterone replacement:

- Prostate growth
- Possible increased risk of heart disease
- Hair loss
- Breast growth
- Increased blood count (which could increase the risk of a blood clot)
- Acne
- Testicular shrinkage
- Reduced fertility
- Worsening of sleep apnea

Let's go through these so you can make an informed decision about whether or not testosterone replacement is something that seems right for you.

Prostate health

In the past, doctors were taught that testosterone replacement increases the risk of prostate cancer. Fortunately, we now know that this isn't true, but unfortunately not all doctors got the update, so your doctor may still have some concerns.

Why Can't I Keep Up Anymore?

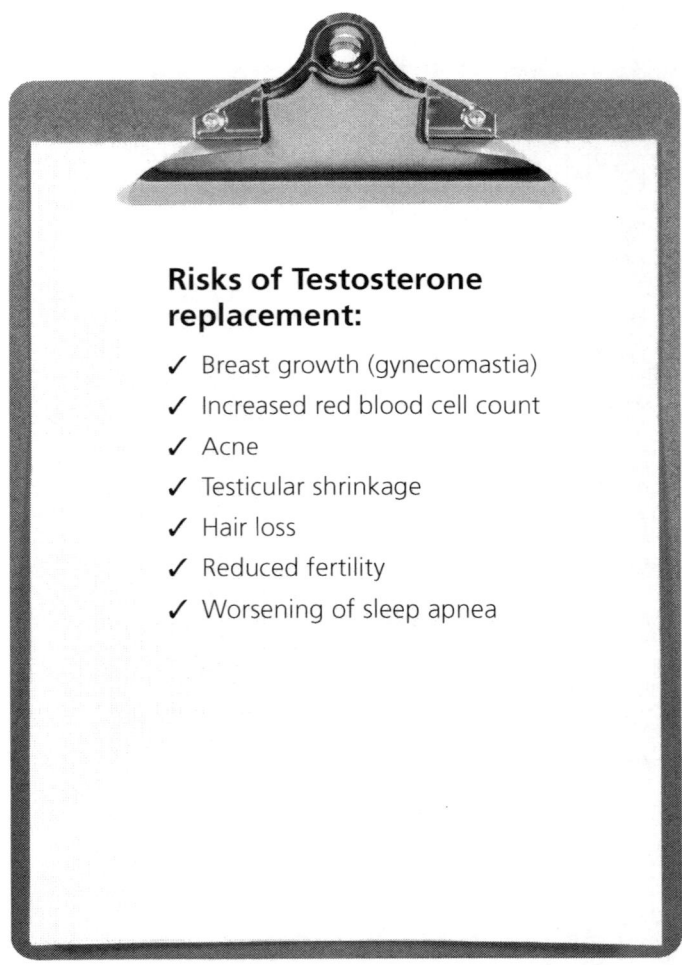

Risks of Testosterone replacement:

- ✓ Breast growth (gynecomastia)
- ✓ Increased red blood cell count
- ✓ Acne
- ✓ Testicular shrinkage
- ✓ Hair loss
- ✓ Reduced fertility
- ✓ Worsening of sleep apnea

Medical Treatment for Low T

Research has actually shown that LOW testosterone, especially paired with higher estrogen, is a risk factor for developing prostate cancer. (2)

Here's where the controversy comes in. We know that if we use treatments to shut down testosterone production, prostate tumors will shrink. The concern is that if we increase your testosterone level, and you have a prostate tumor that we haven't diagnosed yet, the tumor could grow more.

According to Dr Abraham Morgentaler, a board certified Urologist at Harvard, this isn't actually the case. (3) If you want to learn more, I recommend reading his book, Testosterone For Life. He does an excellent job of reviewing this issue.

Doing a screening PSA test (to look for possible prostate cancer) should be done before starting on testosterone replacement therapy. If you currently have prostate cancer, then testosterone treatment is not recommended.

Heart disease controversy

There are thousands of studies looking at the benefits of testosterone (and different forms of testosterone replacement) on heart health. The overwhelming majority of studies show that testosterone is good for men's heart health.

Unfortunately, two studies suggested that testosterone replacement could increase the risk of a heart attack. These studies were widely criticized, and had some problems.

One study looked at the risk of heart disease in men given testosterone replacement. After the fact it was discovered that 10% of the participants in the study were actually women!

Why Can't I Keep Up Anymore?

Nonetheless, the lawyers came out in droves and threatened lawsuits. Many doctors got in trouble with their medical boards if one of their male patients had a heart attack while on testosterone replacement (without actually proving that the testosterone had anything to do with it).

In reviewing the medical literature, the research that supports testosterone for heart health is very large, with many studies over many years. (4)(5)(6) The research suggesting there may be a problem with heart health is based on a tiny number of questionable studies.

Here is my take on the issue: There may be an increased risk of having a heart attack or stroke within the first year of starting testosterone replacement if you have pre-existing heart disease.

If you don't have a problem within the first year, then in time your risk of a heart attack should go down. And since testosterone is good for your heart, it is my medical opinion that for the majority of men the benefits of testosterone outweigh the risks.

Testosterone helps improve blood sugar, lowers inflammation, helps with weight loss, strengthens muscles (including your heart muscle) and improves energy and motivation (which are pretty important for maintaining good lifestyle habits). (7) It also improves sexual function (8) and research shows that men who have more sex have less risk for heart disease (men who have sex at least twice a week have 45% less heart disease than men who have sex only once a month!) (9)

Medical Treatment for Low T

It's possible that living with symptoms of low T because of the fear of having a heart attack may lead to an overall increase in heart attack risk! Please be sure to discuss your individual risks and benefits with your doctor so you can make the best decision.

Estrogen and your heart

A little bit of estrogen is important for men—it helps to prevent bone loss (just like in women) and it's important in heart health. Estrogen in men has not been studied very much. It appears that not enough estrogen is a problem, and too much is a problem too. Just like Goldilocks, it is important for the estrogen level to be "just right".

When estrogen levels are too low, bone loss and heart health are issues. Too much estrogen can contribute to erectile dysfunction. (10) When estrogen levels are too high, men may feel more emotional and "in touch with their feelings". (11) This may not be intrinsically bad, but crying at the movies and becoming irritable and dramatic may not be so desirable for a man.

Years ago, I had a patient who was a high level executive at a bank. Multiple times he found himself on the verge of tears while in meetings with the other bank executives, and had to excuse himself before he started sobbing. This was very startling and worrisome—he had never experienced anything like this before. Once his estrogen level was normalized he got back to feeling like himself again.

Why Can't I Keep Up Anymore?

Hair loss

Boosting testosterone can increase hair loss in men with male pattern baldness. If you have male pattern baldness, your genes cause your hair follicles to be sensitive to dihydrotestosterone, or DHT, which is made out of testosterone. DHT damages the hair follicles, eventually resulting in hair loss, typically in the frontal areas and crown of your head. Boosting testosterone will typically increase the level of DHT, which can accelerate hair loss.

There are medications for hair loss, including finasteride (Propecia) and dutasteride (Avodart), which work by blocking the conversion of testosterone to DHT. Taking a low dose of finasteride can help here, but may also diminish some of the benefits of testosterone therapy! Most concerning is that a small percentage of men who take one of these medications find they have a dramatic reduction in sex drive (12), which may not come back even after stopping the medicine!

This can be a tough one for many men. Do you worry about keeping your hair, at the expense of your sex life……?

My suggestion if you are worried about hair loss is to use saw palmetto (which is an herbal supplement that helps reduce the conversion of testosterone to DHT) and see if this helps. If you are noting an increase in hair loss, you could try the lowest dose of finasteride.

While the blood level of DHT is not directly correlated with the extent of hair loss, your blood level of DHT should be monitored to make sure that you aren't converting more testosterone to DHT than expected.

Gynecomastia

The dreaded "man boobs". Exactly what you DON'T want. Breast growth can be seen on testosterone therapy if the estrogen level goes too high. It happens over time, and monitoring estrogen levels can prevent this. In 13 years of prescribing testosterone I have never had this happen to a patient.

If you think you are noticing a growth in breast tissue starting, it's very important to notify your doctor and have your estrogen level tested as soon as possible. Don't let it go on too long, because the breast growth may not be reversible even with stopping testosterone or reducing your estrogen level.

Some men have what appears to be an increase in breast size due to weight gain. If it is simply fat deposits and not actual growth of breast tissue, this will resolve with weight loss.

Blood "thickening"

Erythrocytosis is the medical term for a high red blood cell count. Testosterone stimulates your bone marrow to make more red blood cells. This is why men typically have a higher red blood cell level than women.

The concern is that testosterone therapy can sometimes make your red blood cell level go higher than normal. This is kind of like "thickening" your blood. We generally like a little bit of blood thinning—this is why some doctors recommend taking a baby aspirin—to "thin" the blood and reduce the risk of a blood clot. We worry that if your blood is "thicker" that there could be an increase in the risk of blood clots.

Erythrocytosis is more commonly seen in testosterone injections (13), probably because the small spikes in testosterone after an injection trigger the bone marrow more. Sometimes changing to a different route (such as pellets or topical cream or gel) can help. Lowering the dose of testosterone can help.

Another solution to this problem is donating blood regularly (for example every three months or so). You're doing something good for your community (and possibly lowering your risk of a blood clot). If you are not a candidate for donating blood, you can have what we call a 'therapeutic phlebotomy'—they take your blood, but throw it out.

Acne

Testosterone can trigger acne in some men. This isn't something that we see very often in men on testosterone replacement, but it is possible. Addressing gut health and skin health in other ways can help, and lowering the dose should help.

Testicular atrophy

When you are on testosterone replacement, the pituitary gland no longer needs to release LH to stimulate the testes, and the cells in the testes no longer have to work to make testosterone. As a result the size of the testes can get smaller.

Medical Treatment for Low T

Young men at the gym taking extremely large doses of testosterone can have very significant testicular shrinkage. Even men on physiologic doses (meaning your testosterone level is in the upper half of the normal range, not three times above the normal range!) have some testicular shrinkage. Some men don't even really notice, but this is something that is quite upsetting to others.

If this is a problem for you, there are treatments that can be added to help. Clomiphene is a pill that can be taken once or twice a week to tell the pituitary to release some LH after all. HCG (human chorionic gonadotropin) acts like LH and directly stimulates the testes. It is given as a tiny injection 2-3 times a week. Both of these work well to reverse testicular shrinkage.

Fertility issues

When men take testosterone replacement, the cells that make sperm can be shut down, and sperm count can drop. Being on testosterone can't be considered birth control, but a man wanting to add to his family should think carefully about testosterone replacement.

On the other hand, HCG and clomiphene described previously can be used. They are routinely used in male fertility treatments to stimulate sperm production. So if you use them to boost testosterone levels, you will also be boosting sperm production (instead of turning it off).

Why Can't I Keep Up Anymore?

Sleep apnea

Testosterone replacement can worsen sleep apnea. Since sleep apnea is one of the causes of low testosterone, if you have been diagnosed with low T and have a suspicion that you could have sleep apnea, this should be evaluated and treated. Some of the symptoms of sleep apnea overlap with symptoms of low T. If you don't address your sleep apnea, you are unlikely to feel as good as you expect even if you start testosterone replacement.

Common symptoms of sleep apnea include:
- Loud snoring
- Waking up with a choking or gasping sensation
- Sleepiness during the day
- Memory problems
- Mood problems
- Weight gain
- Stopping breathing in the night (you'll have to ask your bed partner if you do this)

As with anything, testosterone replacement has risks and benefits. For most men, the benefits of testosterone replacement outweigh the risks, but it is important to talk to your doctor about your personal history and risk factors.

CHAPTER 7

Lifestyle Changes For Optimal Health

Whether or not you choose to go on testosterone replacement, improving your lifestyle habits is one thing that's really non-negotiable. If you do end up on testosterone replacement, putting testosterone into a healthy body will help you get the best results and minimize side effects.

I feel very passionately that if you want to live a high performance life you're going to have to treat your body like a high performance vehicle.

Taking vitamin supplements or testosterone replacement can only go so far. They can never make up for poor lifestyle habits.

5 Steps for Healthy Nutrition

There is a lot of confusion about healthy nutrition. One day you'll hear an expert say, "You need to be vegan." The next day it's paleo or keto or something else.

Why Can't I Keep Up Anymore?

One day eggs are good, the next they are bad. (Don't listen—eggs are good!).

This isn't a book about nutrition, but here are two important points:

1. There is no one perfect diet for everyone. It is probably true that some people will be healthier on a vegan diet without any animal products, and others will be healthier on a keto diet, which is high in healthy fats. All of these different diets have some good things about them. Instead of getting hung up on what proportion of each type of food to eat, it is much more important to follow point #2.

2. The quality of food that you eat is the most important part of your diet. Eating processed food is unhealthy whether you are vegan or paleo or keto or whatever. If you are eating healthy whole food, in the form it is found in nature, then how much animal food you eat (or don't eat) or how much fat or carbs or whatever becomes less important.

You've probably heard the saying, "If you can't say it, don't eat it."

Here are some other fun tips from one of my favorite health writers, Michael Pollan, to make the point:

- "If it came from a plant, eat it; if it was made in a plant, don't."

Lifestyle Changes for Optimal Health

- "Don't eat anything your great-grandmother wouldn't recognize as food."
- "Don't eat breakfast cereals that change the color of the milk." (I know you already know that but it makes me laugh…)

Here are five basic tips for healthy nutrition (that work no matter what nutrition program you are following)

1. Avoid sugar. Sugar is a toxin. It causes inflammation and contributes to chronic disease. I find that most of my patients think that they don't eat a lot of sugar, but they don't realize how much hidden sugar is in the foods that they are eating. Things like ketchup, BBQ sauce, salad dressing, fruit yogurt, granola bars, and orange juice are loaded with sugar and it all adds up.

2. Read labels. If you avoid processed foods like these, your sugar intake will automatically go down.

3. Eat more fruits and veggies. Again, a lot of my patients tell me that they think they are eating a good amount of fruit and veggies. But when we dig into it, they are getting only a couple of servings a day.

    While that is certainly a lot better than nothing, the recommendation is to get 7-10 servings a day, with the majority coming from veggies (and for our conversation, as my kids are used to hearing at our dinner table, corn and potatoes don't count).

Why Can't I Keep Up Anymore?

The goal is to fill at least half of your plate with vegetables and eat veggies of all different colors, because the colors contain the antioxidants and other nutrients that are so beneficial to your health.

4. Eat fat. Yes, that's right; we WANT you to eat fat. Yay! The days of bland, boring low fat diets are over. It turns out that we were wrong when we told you that fat was bad for you.

    The important point is that it has to be HEALTHY fats. Deep fried foods, hot dogs, baloney, and onion rings are still not good for you. But there are lots of delicious healthy fats that make food taste better and help you feel full, while improving your health!

    Examples of good fats (that we want you to eat) are nuts, seeds (like ground flax seeds, chia seeds, hemp seeds and raw pumpkin seeds), olive oil, avocado and avocado oil, coconut and coconut oil. Even butter can be okay, but look for organic butter.

    Your brain is largely made of fat! My kids used to like call each other 'fat head'. ("But mom! It's the truth!") Many of your hormones, including testosterone, are made from cholesterol. If you want healthy hormones and a healthy brain, a low fat diet is not the best choice.

    On the other hand, trans fats are bad for your brain and for your hormones. Trans fats are man-made 'franken-fats' that promote disease. They are found in

Lifestyle Changes for Optimal Health

margarine, shortening, commercially prepared baked goods, and deep fryers, so please steer clear of these foods.

5. Choose the best quality animal protein you can get. If you choose to be vegetarian, just skip this one. I generally don't advise people that they need to give up all animal protein, but it is true that the standard meat eaten by most Americans is not healthful.

    Beef from feed lots (where the cows are fed grain, given antibiotics, and pumped with steroids) is not a great idea. But eating grass fed/grass finished beef occasionally is probably fine. Look for pastured eggs, free range chickens, and wild caught fish.

    Try to lean more towards animals with fewer legs: cows and pigs have four legs, chicken and turkey have two legs, and fish and eggs have none. Fill your plate with veggies and use the protein as the condiment or side dish, instead of the other way around.

6. Watch the starchy carbs. Different nutrition programs recommend restricting carbs more or less, but what is generally agreed upon is that a high processed carb diet is the recipe for diabetes.

    A low carb diet is a good idea if you have a blood sugar problem or are trying to lose weight. Even if you aren't going to go on a low carb diet, too many carbs is not a good idea. A high carb meal causes your blood sugar to spike, which affects insulin and cortisol, which both cause weight gain and lower testosterone levels.

Exercise

I know. Not everyone loves to exercise. But if you want to treat your body like a high performance vehicle, exercise is critical.

The type of exercise that you do matters. It's not necessary to spend hours every day in the gym. In fact, if you do spend hours every day in the gym (especially if you are really competitive and working out hard) you are probably over-exercising, which makes cortisol go up. High cortisol breaks down your muscle and works against you. Instead, work smarter.

Resistance exercise (muscle building) helps boost your testosterone level, and is even more important than cardio. If you are working out multiple muscle groups by going from exercise to exercise with less rest, then you're raising your heart rate and getting some cardio benefits anyway.

Have you ever looked at a sprinter and a marathoner? Who is strong and muscular and who is very lean and light, with low muscle mass? Long distance endurance exercise typically causes the body to break down some of the protein in your muscles to use as fuel. This isn't a problem if you run a mile or two, but extreme endurance sports are actually not so healthy.

Lifestyle Changes for Optimal Health

If you want to look good, feel good, and stay healthy then focus on resistance exercise, and throw in some cardio if you want. Three good workouts a week for 20 minutes to an hour should be enough.

Stress

When you are stressed cortisol goes up, which causes testosterone to go down, so managing stress in a healthy way is important. The truth is it's not about how much stress you have but about how you allow the stress to affect you. So even if you can't change your circumstances, you can change how you react.

Some healthy ways of reducing the effects of stress on your body include:

- Yoga
- Breathing exercises
- Meditation
- Mindfulness
- Being outside in nature
- Petting your dog
- Laughter
- Heartfelt prayer
- Visualization

Incorporate several of these into your daily routine. If this is kind of new to you and you're having trouble getting started, download one of the many apps to help. Calm and

InSight Timer are examples, but there are many. They have guided meditations, breathing exercises, and other tools to help you get started (and they're free to get started!)

If you are a type A, driven, competitive, person, then you will typically have a hard time with this.

It's hard to take time out of your day to 'just breathe' (there are so many other things that you could be getting accomplished with that time). And trying to "turn off your brain" can be hard and annoying. But this is VERY important (you know I'm talking to you...).

Type A people need this the most and can benefit the most. If you're type A, you CAN accomplish this if you just decide that you are going to make it a priority. Commit to trying something for a week (breathing exercises are the easiest) and see how it goes.

Exercise also counts as a stress reliever (unless you are highly competitive, in which case it could be a stressor instead) but don't underestimate the power of mindfulness and breathing.

Sleep

You make testosterone at night during sleep. If you aren't getting enough good quality sleep, then you are probably not doing the best job at making testosterone. Sleep is also important for your immune system function, your weight, your blood sugar balance, your mood, and so much more. In fact, we can take healthy college students, deprive them of sleep for a few nights, and watch their blood sugar levels start to rise.

Lifestyle Changes for Optimal Health

Men who have sleep apnea have an increased risk of low T. This is probably partly due to the fact they aren't getting good quality sleep, and likely also because the underlying factors that contribute to sleep apnea (like being overweight) are the same things that predispose you to having low T.

If you think you snore and could be at risk of sleep apnea, please have a sleep study done to find out for sure. If you do have sleep apnea, proper treatment is important if you want to be healthy. Sleep apnea doesn't just increase your risk for low T, it also increases your risk for high blood pressure, heart disease, and many other chronic conditions you don't want.

Alcohol

Alcohol is not good for your liver, and your hormones are processed in your liver. This is why alcoholics with liver disease typically have high estrogen levels.

If you want to be optimally healthy and have healthy hormone levels, then you'll need to keep your alcohol intake in check. Generally the guidelines are 1-2 drinks/day for men (and that doesn't mean you can save them up and have 10 on Friday night!).

If you don't drink much alcohol now, I don't generally recommend drinking on purpose for your health. While a little red wine may be good for your heart, it is not good for cancer risks or hormone health. If you love Bourbon, it's okay to have a glass, but otherwise save it for special occasions.

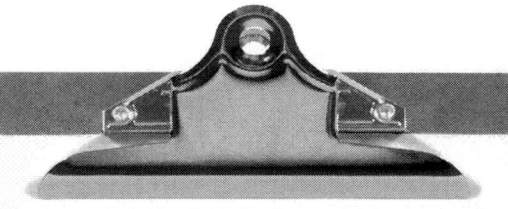

Lifestyle changes:

✓ Nutrition
- · Avoid sugar
- · Increase fruits and veggies
- · Add healthy fats
- · Choose high quality protein
- · Watch the starchy carbs

✓ Exercise

✓ Stress management

✓ Reduce alcohol

✓ Sleep

CHAPTER 8

Supplements for Men's Health

Taking vitamins will not make up for an unhealthy diet. But adding certain supplements can give you an edge and help to optimize your health. These are my top recommendations for supplements to support men's health, but in my office I prefer to do a lab evaluation to find out exactly what vitamins you need based on the results.

Vitamin D

Did you know that vitamin D isn't really a vitamin, it's actually a hormone! It is made in your skin in response to sunlight. But in our modern world, our bodies are not making adequate amounts of vitamin D.

It's extremely rare for me to see someone with an optimal D level if they are not taking a supplement. Even if you golf or play tennis regularly and have a great tan, you may be surprised that your vitamin D level isn't optimal.

Why Can't I Keep Up Anymore?

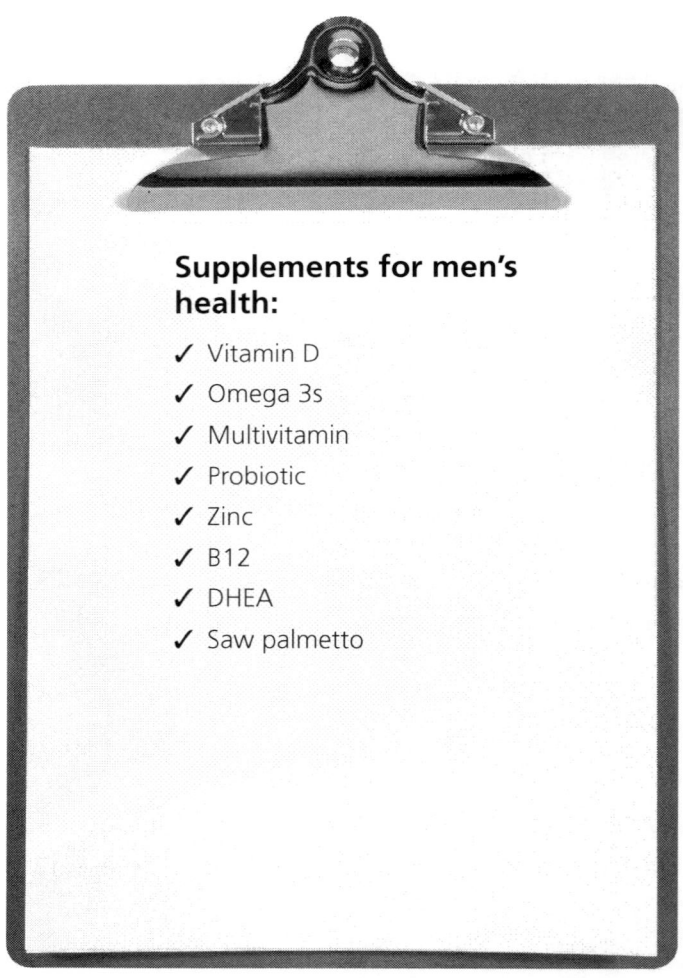

Supplements for men's health:
- ✓ Vitamin D
- ✓ Omega 3s
- ✓ Multivitamin
- ✓ Probiotic
- ✓ Zinc
- ✓ B12
- ✓ DHEA
- ✓ Saw palmetto

Supplements for Men's Health

Vitamin D has a lot of really important roles. It helps your body absorb calcium from your food, so it's important for your teeth and bones. It's also important for healthy blood sugar metabolism and for weight loss. I find that people with low vitamin D have a harder time losing weight, and can be more successful once their level is optimized. (1)

One of the most important jobs of vitamin D is to regulate your immune system. (2) Your immune system is your first line of defense against cancer. We all have stray cancer cells in our bodies, and your immune system should find those cells and get rid of them before they have a chance to cause a problem.

If your vitamin D level is not optimal, your immune system doesn't do a good job and your risk of cancer is increased. (3) Many cancers have been found to be more common with low vitamin D levels, including breast cancer, pancreatic cancer, melanoma and colon cancer.

Vitamin D also turns your genes off and on. We were taught in grade school that you were born with your genes and there is nothing that you can do about it. Now we understand that your genes are constantly getting 'turned off' and 'turned on'. Food is more than calories and energy—food contains information that tells your genes whether to turn off or on. Healthy food turns the helpful genes on and the unhelpful ones off. And this is exactly what vitamin D does, as well. There are some genes that help cancer cells, and vitamin D turns many of these genes off. Some genes help prevent cancer and vitamin D tends to turn these ones on.

Why Can't I Keep Up Anymore?

The "normal" range of vitamin D is controversial. Some labs say 20-80ng/mL, but most labs say 30-100ng/mL. The "optimal" range is also very controversial. If the normal range is 30-100, the half way point is 65, so I suggest aiming for a level midrange, about 60-80. Research suggests that your vitamin D level needs to be above 55 to get the anti-cancer benefits.

Ask your doctor to measure your vitamin D level. They will typically be happy if your level is within the 'normal range,' but look at your actual number. If it is only in the 30s or 40s, consider taking 2000IU vitamin D3 daily. If your level is below 30, take 5000IU daily.

It is important to have your level rechecked in a few months to make sure that it has gone up above 55 (and that it hasn't gone up too high). If you take vitamin D and your level goes up nicely, and then you stop taking it, your level will gradually go back down.

Omega 3

Omega 3 fatty acids are very important nutrients that most people don't get enough of in their diet.

You can get omega 3s from cold water fatty fish such as salmon, but it is imperative to buy wild caught salmon. Farm-raised salmon and other fish like tilapia and catfish are fed "fish chow" instead of their natural diet, so they don't have very much omega 3s.

You can also get omega 3s in plant foods, such as walnuts and flax, but most people aren't very good at converting the

Supplements for Men's Health

type of omega 3s in these foods to the type your body needs, so it's hard to get enough from plants alone.

You can have your omega 3 level checked. I typically measure an omega 3 index, which looks at a variety of omegas including omega 3, 6, and 9, as well as trans fats (which are manmade fats that are very harmful to your health). The omega 3 index evaluates what percentage of your cell membranes is made up of omega 3s. Different labs have different normal ranges, but the goal is to be in the optimal range for your lab.

Omega 3s are used to make up your cell membranes. They keep your cell membrane flexible so that nutrients can get into the cells and waste products can get out. Your hormone receptors are embedded in your cell membrane, so a healthy, flexible membrane allows your hormone receptors to work properly.

When you are deficient in omega 3s (and especially if you have too much trans fats from deep fried food, margarine, and shortening like Crisco) your cell membranes will be stiff—nutrients can't get in, waste products can't get out, and your hormone receptors won't work properly. If you want healthy hormone balance and healthy cells, optimal omega 3 levels are important.

Eat wild caught fatty fish at least a couple of times a week (avoiding the ones highest in mercury like swordfish and tuna) and consider taking a fish oil supplement.

Not all fish oil is created equal so it is important to use a good quality, pharmaceutical grade product. You also need to take a big enough dose to do any good. It is not enough to look at the front label, where it often says "1200mg of fish oil". I don't care how much fish oil is in the capsule, I care about how much omega 3s are in the fish oil. You'll need to turn the bottle around and read the ingredients: look for how many milligrams of EPA and how many milligrams of DHA are in one capsule (and be aware that the serving size is often two capsules, so you'll need to check that too).

EPA+DHA added together should be a minimum of 1000mg daily if you are just trying to maintain good health, and 4000mg daily if you have aches and pains, arthritis, dry eyes, or any kind of neurological problem like Parkinson's.

Most good quality supplements have about 500mg in one capsule, so you may need to take a few capsules (and be warned—fish oil capsules often seem like big horse pills). If you find swallowing the pills a challenge, you can get liquid fish oil (they make ones that don't taste fishy), and you can usually get a good dose in about a tablespoon daily (read the bottle to figure out how much you need to get the dose you want).

Another problem with fish oil capsules is that some people get "fish burps" that are pretty unpleasant. To avoid this, make sure you have a good quality fish oil supplement. You can get enteric coated supplements that are much less likely to "repeat" on you.

Another trick is to keep your fish oil in the freezer! If you swallow a frozen capsule, it will get farther down your digestive tract before the capsule bursts open, so you are much less likely to have digestive problems. The only hard part is you have to remember to open the freezer and take them! (Sometimes they end up "out of sight, out of mind"...)

You should keep the capsules in the fridge anyway after the bottle is opened to keep them fresh and prevent them from going rancid (which will definitely increase the chance of a fish burp!). If your fish oil is old, throw it out and buy something new.

Multivitamin

Taking a multivitamin is another thing that the health care industry has created confusion about.

It seems pretty logical that your body needs all sorts of different nutrients to allow your cells to function properly. It seems reasonable that you should be able to get the nutrients that you need from food.

Unfortunately, our reality is that the food available to us today is very different than the food even 40 years ago. Most food is highly processed and really doesn't contain many healthy nutrients. Even if you do a good job eating fruits and veggies, the soil they are grown in is depleted in nutrients, so the food may not have as much of the vitamins and minerals as we would expect.

Optimal nutrition is critical for health, but medical doctors are simply not trained in nutrition. I had a grand total two hours of lectures on nutrition in medical school, and they were just talking about children with extreme starvation due to famine—not something that is likely contributing to your current health issues.

Why Can't I Keep Up Anymore?

The reality is that most Americans are over-fed and under-nourished. Most of us have nutrient deficiencies! They are typically not severe enough to cause immediate symptoms of a vitamin deficiency, but over time they contribute to our epidemic of chronic disease. If you want to take care of yourself and stay healthy, then nutrition should be important to you.

Of course it's important to eat healthy food (no pill can every replace good nutrition!). But taking a pharmaceutical grade multivitamin is just added insurance to make sure you are getting the vitamins and minerals your body needs.

The tricky part (and the part that has confused medical doctors) is that it needs to be the right kind of multivitamin. In medical studies, they typically just ask people, "Are you taking a multivitamin?" And then, "Have you had a heart attack?" or, "Have you been diagnosed with cancer?" etc. The numbers are crunched to see if the people who said they take a multivitamin have had less heart attacks or whatever diseases they have on their checklist.

Usually they don't find any difference. But here's the thing: if you walk into a standard pharmacy or your grocery store and grab whatever brand of multivitamin is available, you are likely wasting your time and money. The multi most likely contains synthetic versions of many of the vitamins, the minerals are almost certainly in the form that is not well absorbed, and they have probably added food coloring and other filler ingredients. So, it's not really fair to expect they're going to do much good for your health.

Here are a few things to check on your multivitamin to

determine if it's worth taking or should be chucked in the trash. If it contains any of these, toss it.

Synthetic Vitamin E—In the small print on the back of the bottle, look for dl-alpha tocopherol. This is the synthetic form that you DON'T want. Instead look for d-alpha tocopherol. Did you catch the difference? dl—is the synthetic version. d—is the natural version. Such a tiny difference, but it is important.

Folic Acid—This is also a manmade vitamin. In nature you get folinic acid or folate, but folic acid is cheap and readily available. Most medical doctors (myself included) were never taught that the form of the vitamin is important. You should look for folinic acid or methylfolate (which is the activated form of folate).

Cyanocobalamin—This is not the best form of Vit B12, but it is definitely the most common. Look for methylcobalamin, which is the neurologically activated form of B12.

Calcium carbonate—This is an inexpensive form of calcium, but it is poorly absorbed. Calcium citrate is a better choice. My preferred form of calcium is calcium hydroxyapatite (also called MCHC), but you will only find this at a health food store.

Magnesium oxide—This is another inexpensive form of magnesium that is not well absorbed. There are a lot of better choices, including magnesium glycinate, malate, or citrate. There are even more forms, but let's keep it simple—skip the "oxide" (you can remember because it's the one with the X) and anything else will be ok.

Two other things to watch for:

Food coloring—Often it will say 'FD&C Red #40' or something similar. Do you care what color your vitamin is? No self-respecting nutraceutical company would ever add food coloring to their products.

Sugar—I don't feel like I should really have to mention this one. If your vitamin has sugar (or sucrose, glucose, fructose, or anything similar) that should be a huge red flag. Just toss it and find something better.

Look for a pharmaceutical grade multivitamin at a health food store or online. The big box chain stores, pharmacies, and grocery stores are generally not a good place to purchase nutritional supplements.

Unless you have been diagnosed with low iron, it is generally advised that men take a multivitamin that does not contain iron. Too much iron is a problem for men, so don't add to the problem with your multivitamin.

Probiotics

We all have trillions of bacteria in our gut, and it turns out that those bacteria are very important to our health. You need the right ones to help you digest your food, keep your colon cells healthy, make some of your vitamins, and regulate your immune system. When your gut microbiome is imbalanced, this contributes to many chronic health issues. There is an explosion of research into this area, and we are learning more at a tremendous pace. The health of your microbiome also affects your hormone health.

Testosterone is converted into estrogen and too much estrogen is a problem for men. Estrogen is dumped into your gut by your liver, and it gets pooped out. If you are constipated, then the estrogen has more of a chance to get reabsorbed back into your system and cause problems. Also, when you don't have the right balance of gut bugs you can end up with too much of something called beta-glucuronidase, which reabsorbs more estrogen back into your body.

The bottom line is if you want to have optimal health, including optimal hormone health, and if you want to get the best results from your hormone therapy with minimal risks, then you need to have balanced gut bugs. Taking a probiotic can help.

Choosing a probiotic can be tricky. Once again, the grocery store or big box store is not the best place to look. Look for a supplement that has a minimum of 15 billion organisms/capsule and contains at least a couple of different strains. Most commonly you will see bifidobacter and acidophilus.

If you have digestive symptoms like diarrhea, constipation, irritable bowel syndrome, gastroesophageal reflux (heartburn), or indigestion, taking a supplement may not fix the whole problem. You may require a more thorough evaluation by a Functional Medicine practitioner.

Please be aware that your gut health is important, and these are signals from your body that something is not right inside. Functional Medicine has a lot to offer to help optimize your gut health. Taking an antacid is not fixing the problem; it's just putting a Band-Aid over the symptoms.

Zinc

Zinc is important in the production of testosterone (4) and for a healthy prostate. It is also important for immune system function, mood, and many other things! You can request your zinc level be tested in a blood test, but this is not typically done so your doctor may not be willing. You can take a zinc supplement with 15-50mg daily. If you are taking a multivitamin, it will likely have a small amount of zinc already.

B12

This important vitamin helps with energy, metabolism, and mood (which are all things that go south with low T). If your Vit B12 levels are low, you won't get full symptom resolution even on testosterone replacement. This is a common blood test to order, and it shouldn't be hard to get your doctor to order it for you.

B12 can be hard to absorb in your stomach, so pills aren't the best option to boost B12 levels. Sublingual drops or lozenges, which dissolve under your tongue, are readily available and preferable. A typical dose is 1000mg daily.

Look for methylcobalamin (which is the neurologically active form) instead of cyanocobalamin (which is the more common form but may not work as well for everyone).

DHEA

DHEA is a hormone that your body can use to make testosterone and in the U.S. it is available as an over-the-counter supplement. I recommend having your DHEA level tested before taking this. It would be a waste of money (and possibly could cause side effects) if you take this when your DHEA level is already normal or high. (Finding highish DHEA levels in men is not uncommon).

Unfortunately, when men take DHEA it is much more likely to convert into estrogen than testosterone. It usually results in only a modest increase in testosterone (some studies have shown about a 13% increase), but a significant increase in estrogen—which doesn't really allow for proper hormone balance.

While taking DHEA is not likely going to restore testosterone levels, there are some important reasons to consider taking DHEA if your level is low. As an androgen hormone, DHEA helps support blood sugar metabolism, immune system function, sense of vitality, muscle and bone health, and it is needed to be able to make enough growth hormone.

A typical dose for men is 25-50mg daily. It is important to measure and follow your DHEA level. Since DHEA tends to convert into estrogen, it's also important to follow your estrogen level to make sure it doesn't rise too much.

Why Can't I Keep Up Anymore?

Saw palmetto

This herb is native to the southern United States. It has been used for hair loss, urinary tract health and prostate health.(5) Saw palmetto inhibits the enzyme 5 alpha reductase which converts testosterone to DHT. DHT is the hormone implicated in male pattern baldness, so saw palmetto may help minimize hair loss. DHT also stimulate prostate growth. Saw palmetto works like a natural version of finasteride (Proscar or Propecia) or dustateride (Avodart), which are medications often used for preventing hair loss and for urinary problems caused by an enlarged prostate.

Other supplements that may support men's sexual health:

Yohimbine—This is a nutritional supplement from the bark of the West African yohimbe tree which has been used as an aphrodisiac and for ED. The science shows mixed results. (6) Use caution with this supplement if you are on blood thinner medications or have heart problems.

Deer Antler Velvet—This is just what it sounds like—the velvet from a male deer. It has been used for centuries to help increase strength and immunity. Studies in rats show that it increases testosterone and improves sexual performance in older rats (7), but we don't have human studies to back this up. Antler velvet contains IGF-1, which controls human growth hormone levels in your body. Some athletes have tried using deer antler velvet to increase sports performance, but the studies have been mixed. Interestingly, antlers are the fastest growing organs in any mammal, and it is thought that the IGF-1 in the velvet is important for fueling that rapid growth.

Stinging Nettle—this herb contains an ingredient called beta sitosterol that has been used by Greeks, Romans and Native Americans for healthy prostates and erectile function. It binds to sex hormone binding globulin (SHBG) to increase free testosterone. (8) There are no human studies to prove that stinging nettle helps with ED.

Horny Goat Weed (epimedium)—This is a traditional Chinese remedy for low libido and erectile function. Studies in rats suggest the herb may help increase blood flow to the penis. (9)

Tribulus terestris—This herb may boost libido and may help improve erectile function according to some studies, although the exact mechanism of action is still being investigated. (10)

Arginine

Arginine is a naturally occurring amino acid that can help with erectile function. It also helps trigger release of human growth hormone, which is the hormone of youth and vitality.

Why Can't I Keep Up Anymore?

It works best when combined with another amino acid, called citrulline. (11, 12)

Unfortunately, most men I've talked to have not had marked improvement in their sexual symptoms with these supplements. Other than Yohimbine, there is fairly low risk in trying them. It's always best to discuss use of supplements with your doctor, but please understand that western medical schools do not have courses on the pros and cons of things like "horny goat weed" and "deer antler velvet."

If your testosterone level is normal, cleaning up your lifestyle habits may be all you need. Trying these supplements may be reasonable.

If your testosterone level is low, you may feel a lot better with testosterone replacement.

Supplements for Men's Health

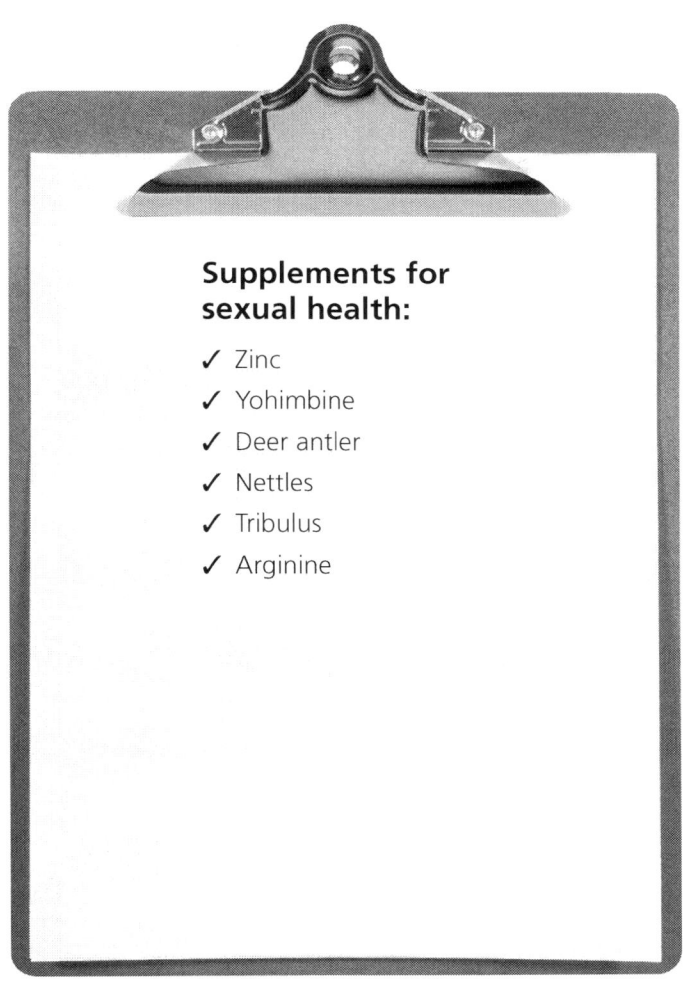

Supplements for sexual health:

- ✓ Zinc
- ✓ Yohimbine
- ✓ Deer antler
- ✓ Nettles
- ✓ Tribulus
- ✓ Arginine

CHAPTER 9

Stressed Out: Cortisol and Your Health

Does this sound like you?

The alarm goes off, and you press snooze (a couple of times) before you're able to rouse yourself enough to get out of bed. Even after you drag your body upright, your brain is still not fully online, and you need a jolt of caffeine to help you feel completely human.

Once you finally get yourself going, you're okay for a while, until the bewitching time, between 2-4 p.m. when your energy crashes. In order to make it through until dinnertime, you need more caffeine or sugar (or a power nap!)

You feel a little better after supper, but early in the evening you sit on the couch and feel drowsy. It's only 7:30 p.m. (too early to go to bed!) If you stay up late enough, you get a second wind! Now at 10 p.m. your brain feels more alert, and sometimes you end up getting your best work of the day done at night.

Why Can't I Keep Up Anymore?

The problem is that even when you force yourself to go to bed, your brain is wide awake (despite being tired most of the day) and now you can't fall asleep! When you finally fall asleep, you end up waking up at 2 a.m. and 4 a.m., so you don't get good quality sleep. And then there's that darn alarm again!

If you can relate to some of this, you certainly aren't alone! This is really common in our modern society, but it's not normal. It could be a sign of a cortisol problem.

Cortisol is your main stress hormone—it's kind of like "long acting adrenaline".

Here's how things are supposed to work: If you have a sudden stressful experience, like running late for an important appointment and getting stuck in traffic, your cortisol level goes up to help you cope with the stress. Then when you get there and everything turns out okay, your cortisol level goes back down to normal. This is a normal stress response.

In the past, our stresses were physical things like being chased by a saber-toothed tiger and having to run for our life. The physical activity (running) helped us to clear the extra stress hormones from our system. Today, your stresses typically don't involve running for your life—they are much more likely to involve fuming at the slow traffic while you sit in your car worrying about being late for your appointment. When you experience stress day in and day out, the end result can be chronically elevated cortisol levels.

If your cortisol level remains chronically elevated, health problems can follow.

Stressed Out

High cortisol may promote:

- Feeling "wired but tired"
- Mood symptoms (including depression, anxiety and irritability)
- Food cravings (for salt or sugar)
- Weight gain (especially belly fat!)
- Insomnia
- High blood pressure
- Poor memory (high cortisol shrinks your brain!)
- Weakened immune system (more likely to get sick and take longer to recover)
- Difficulty handling stress
- Feeling tired after exercise
- Loss of interest in things you used to enjoy
- Decreased sex drive
- Loss of muscle mass
- Low testosterone
- Accelerated aging

In a nutshell, high cortisol ages you at an accelerated rate—it is a wear and tear hormone! You've probably witnessed this—people who have lived under extremely stressful conditions often look older than their biological age.

Over time, high cortisol is damaging to your brain. In self defense, your brain may shut down the signals to your adrenal gland. Your cortisol levels may drop inappropriately and now you don't have enough cortisol to get you through the day.

Why Can't I Keep Up Anymore?

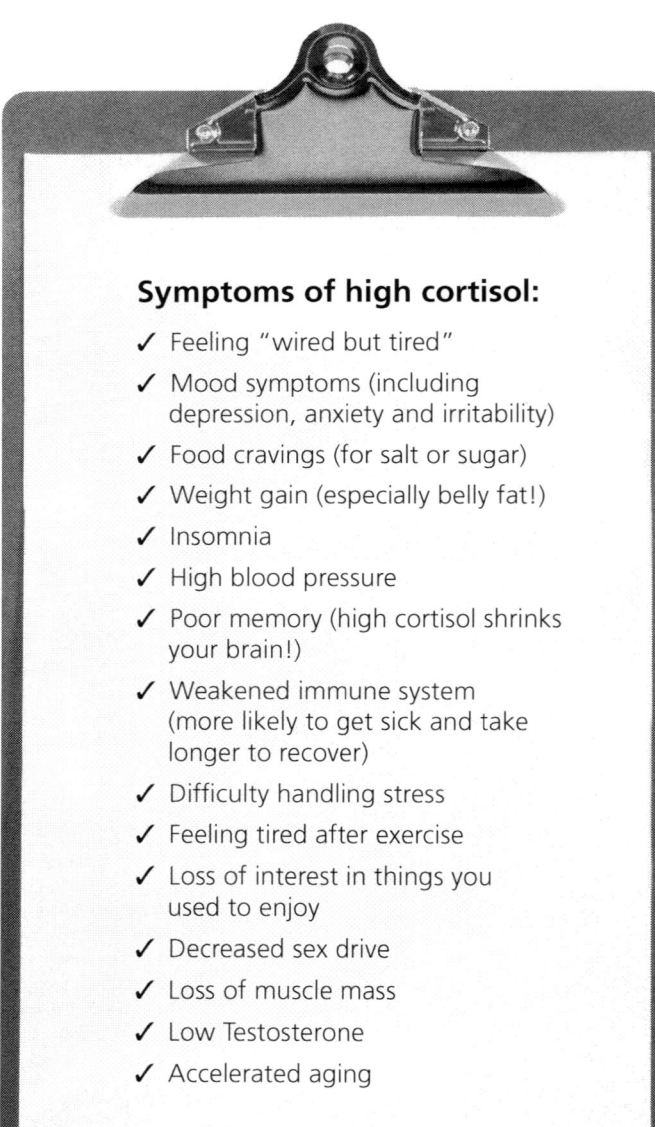

Symptoms of high cortisol:

- ✓ Feeling "wired but tired"
- ✓ Mood symptoms (including depression, anxiety and irritability)
- ✓ Food cravings (for salt or sugar)
- ✓ Weight gain (especially belly fat!)
- ✓ Insomnia
- ✓ High blood pressure
- ✓ Poor memory (high cortisol shrinks your brain!)
- ✓ Weakened immune system (more likely to get sick and take longer to recover)
- ✓ Difficulty handling stress
- ✓ Feeling tired after exercise
- ✓ Loss of interest in things you used to enjoy
- ✓ Decreased sex drive
- ✓ Loss of muscle mass
- ✓ Low Testosterone
- ✓ Accelerated aging

Stressed Out

This is when things get even worse: you start to feel really exhausted, burned out, have difficulty coping with life, and little things (that shouldn't really be stressful) feel overwhelming.

Symptoms of low cortisol include:

- Feeling tired for no obvious reason
- Feeling overwhelmed and rundown
- Hypoglycemia (drop in blood sugar)
- Digestive problems
- Decreased sex drive
- Low blood pressure
- Nervousness
- Insomnia
- Low body temperature
- Allergies
- Decreased ability to handle stress
- Thin and dry skin
- Hair loss
- Pain in upper back or neck
- Feel better suddenly after a meal
- Memory loss
- Feel unrefreshed in the morning even after adequate sleep
- Cravings for salty or sweet snacks
- Difficulty bouncing back from a cold or illness
- Finally feel more awake and alert in the evening, and then have trouble falling asleep

Why Can't I Keep Up Anymore?

Symptoms of low cortisol include:

- ✓ Feeling tired for no obvious reason
- ✓ Feeling overwhelmed or burned out
- ✓ Hypoglycemia (drop in blood sugar)
- ✓ Digestive problems
- ✓ Decreased sex drive
- ✓ Low blood pressure
- ✓ Nervousness
- ✓ Insomnia
- ✓ Low body temperature
- ✓ Allergies
- ✓ Decreased ability to handle stress
- ✓ Thin and dry skin
- ✓ Hair loss
- ✓ Memory loss
- ✓ Feel unrefreshed in the morning even after adequate sleep
- ✓ Cravings for salty or sweet snacks
- ✓ Difficulty bouncing back from a cold or illness
- ✓ Finally feel more awake and alert in the evening, and then have trouble falling asleep

Stressed Out

Many men come to see me because they think they have a problem with testosterone, and they may! But they very commonly also have a problem with cortisol.

Why hasn't your doctor already diagnosed this?

Unfortunately, cortisol problems usually go undiagnosed. Some people who suffer from the physical effects of stress will go from doctor to doctor and be told that they are just fine. They end up feeling like a hypochondriac, because there are no tangible reasons for feeling a little under the weather or tired or just plain rundown. One reason for this is that these symptoms have become part of everyday life for so many people, that the problems are becoming "normal." But it doesn't have to be this way!

Another big "problem" is that there is no prescription drug to treat this. So even if your doctor was able to recognize that your symptoms are the result of stress, they really have nothing to offer to fix the problem, other than to tell you to reduce your stress levels. (But don't worry—there are things you can do, and we'll talk about them in a minute).

The truth is that medical doctors are trained to look for diseases of the adrenal gland, like Cushing's disease (a tumor where your adrenal glands make way too much cortisol) or Addison's (a disease where your adrenal glands are unable to make enough cortisol). These are life-threatening health issues that are uncommon.

When your adrenal glands aren't broken or diseased, but are having problems keeping up with your chronic stress, we

Why Can't I Keep Up Anymore?

call this adrenal fatigue. This term isn't accepted by many doctors—the only options available are Cushing's, Addison's or "normal".

What is adrenal fatigue?

Your body has a very complex system to recognize and respond to stress—that's important to keep you alive! We call this system the Hypothalamic/Pituitary/Adrenal (or HPA) axis. Parts of your brain (the hypothalamus and pituitary glands) recognize that there is stress/danger/famine and send hormone messages to notify your adrenal glands, which pump out cortisol and adrenaline (and other stress hormones) to keep you alive. Very important when a saber tooth tiger jumps out of the bushes, but not so helpful in traffic. This very complex system can get out of whack when it is overworked—the end result is too much or too little cortisol released, and you don't feel good.

If you eat too much, you can expect your waistline to expand. That's just the expected response to too many calories—your body will store the extra calories as fat and you'll have to punch a new hole in your belt. When you have chronic stress you can expect the system that regulates your stress hormones to be affected. It's just how our bodies try to adapt to all that stress. It's not really a disease, but it's a common problem that has significant effects on how you feel and on your overall health and it can be fixed!

Stressed Out

What causes adrenal fatigue?

The number one factor is chronic stress. The function of your adrenal glands is to help in emergency situations. In those situations, you need to remember two very important things:

1. When the adrenal glands go into fight-or-flight mode, everything else going on in your body is pretty much put on hold. Once the adrenal glands start producing cortisol to combat stress, all other metabolic functions slow down.

   - Less hormones are produced (like testosterone and thyroid)
   - Digestion slows down
   - Less blood flows to your organs, so more is available to your muscles to run for your life

2. This kind of adrenal gland function isn't meant to go on for a prolonged period of time. It is a short-term, rapid-fire, instant response. It is meant to last about as long as a sprint, not a marathon.
   When stress is constant in your life, the system that regulates your adrenal glands, the HPA axis, starts to malfunction.

Why Can't I Keep Up Anymore?

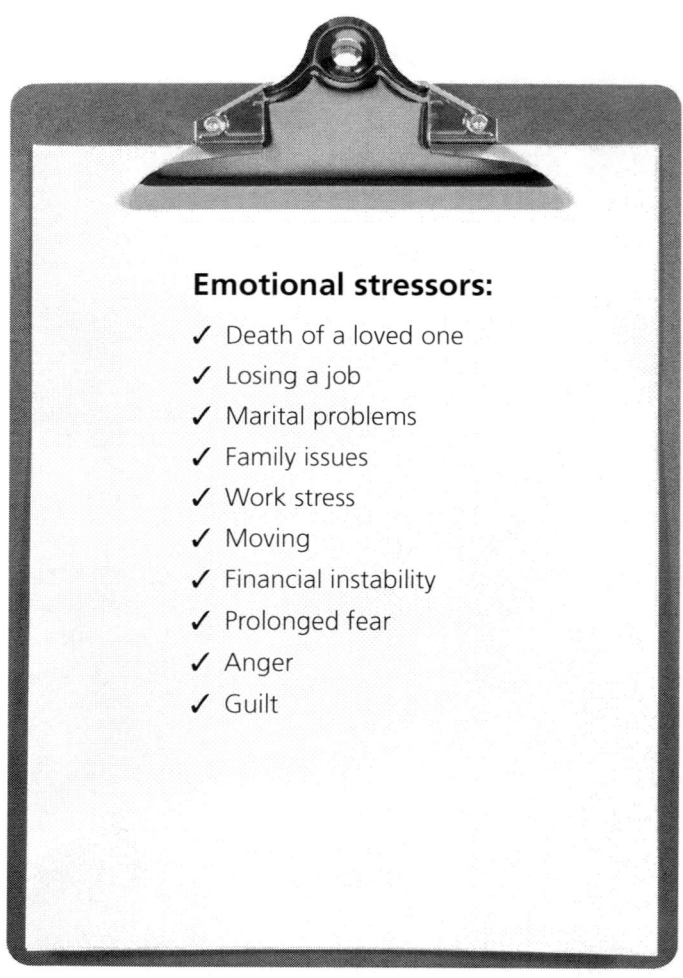

Emotional stressors:
- ✓ Death of a loved one
- ✓ Losing a job
- ✓ Marital problems
- ✓ Family issues
- ✓ Work stress
- ✓ Moving
- ✓ Financial instability
- ✓ Prolonged fear
- ✓ Anger
- ✓ Guilt

Stressed Out

We have many things in life that are stressful:

- Death of a loved one
- Losing a job
- Marital problems
- Family issues
- Work stress
- Moving
- Financial instability
- Prolonged fear
- Anger
- Guilt

When we are thinking about stresses, it is important to realize that there are a lot of things that affect your system besides emotional stress. There are many physical and physiological stresses, as well.

Things like:

- Allergies
- Chronic pain
- Insomnia
- Nutritional deficiencies
- Hormonal imbalances (like low T!)
- Surgery
- Yo-yo dieting
- Infections

Why Can't I Keep Up Anymore?

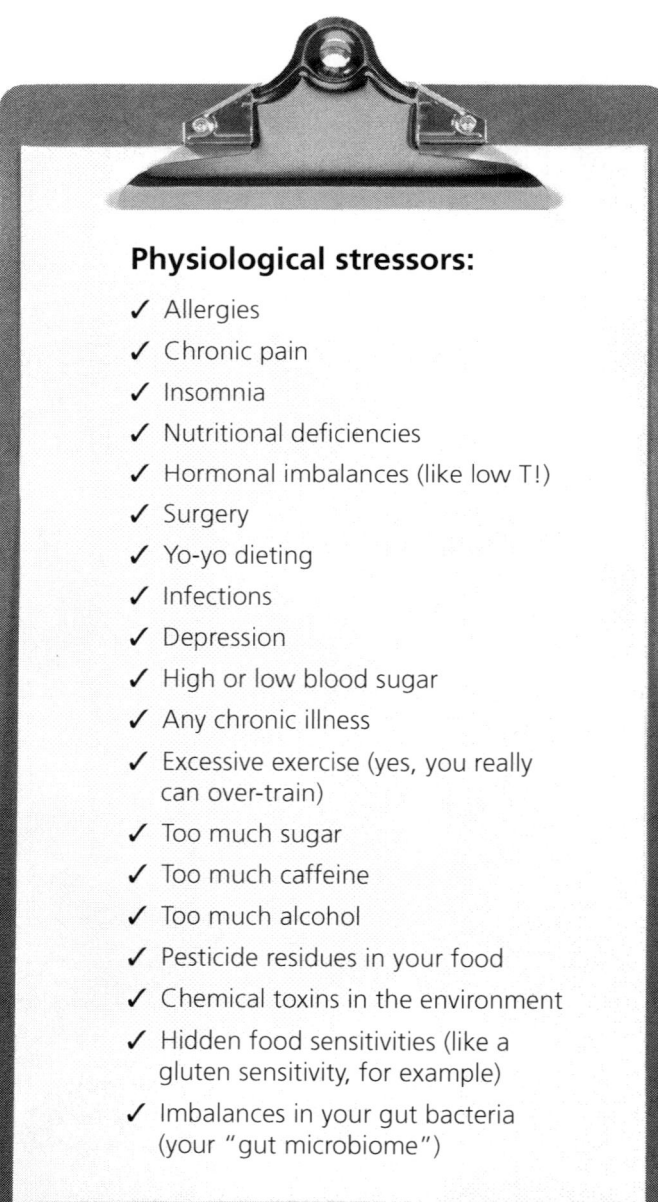

Physiological stressors:

- ✓ Allergies
- ✓ Chronic pain
- ✓ Insomnia
- ✓ Nutritional deficiencies
- ✓ Hormonal imbalances (like low T!)
- ✓ Surgery
- ✓ Yo-yo dieting
- ✓ Infections
- ✓ Depression
- ✓ High or low blood sugar
- ✓ Any chronic illness
- ✓ Excessive exercise (yes, you really can over-train)
- ✓ Too much sugar
- ✓ Too much caffeine
- ✓ Too much alcohol
- ✓ Pesticide residues in your food
- ✓ Chemical toxins in the environment
- ✓ Hidden food sensitivities (like a gluten sensitivity, for example)
- ✓ Imbalances in your gut bacteria (your "gut microbiome")

Stressed Out

- Depression
- High or low blood sugar
- Any chronic illness

Here are some common ones that you may not have considered "stressors":

- Excessive exercise (yes, you really can over-train)
- Too much sugar
- Too much caffeine
- Too much alcohol

You probably also have hidden stresses that you aren't even aware of. Things like:

- Pesticide residues in your food
- Chemical toxins in the environment (like in plastics and cleaning supplies)
- Hidden food sensitivities (like a gluten sensitivity, for example)
- Imbalanced bacteria that live in your intestinal tract (your "gut microbiome")

If you have symptoms of adrenal fatigue, but don't believe that you have a lot of emotional stressors, you may want to look into some of these hidden stressors that could be profoundly affecting your health.

If you add these up, you can see that it's very common in our modern world to have high stress burdens!

Why Can't I Keep Up Anymore?

Why is cortisol so important?

Cortisol is produced by your adrenal glands (they are about the size of a walnut and sit on top of your kidneys). It is one of the only hormones that increases (rather than decreases) as you get older. It is a "wear and tear" hormone—meaning that it accelerates the aging process. On the other hand, testosterone is a "build and repair" hormone that helps to keep your body healthy. So what you DON'T want is high cortisol and low T!

Cortisol has many important functions in the body. (1) It:
- Balances your blood sugar
- Regulates circadian rhythms (helps you sleep at night and be energized in the day)
- Controls weight
- Balances your mood
- Regulates your immune system
- Regulates the other hormones, such as testosterone, estrogen, DHEA, and insulin

How do you know if you really have adrenal fatigue, and you're not just tired and grouchy?

Take a test to find out. Be sure to find a healthcare provider who is knowledgeable about adrenal fatigue. Most understand what to do if the adrenal gland is completely shot (like Cushing's and Addison's, which are rare), but few assess the stages before complete failure.

Cortisol is produced in different amounts at different

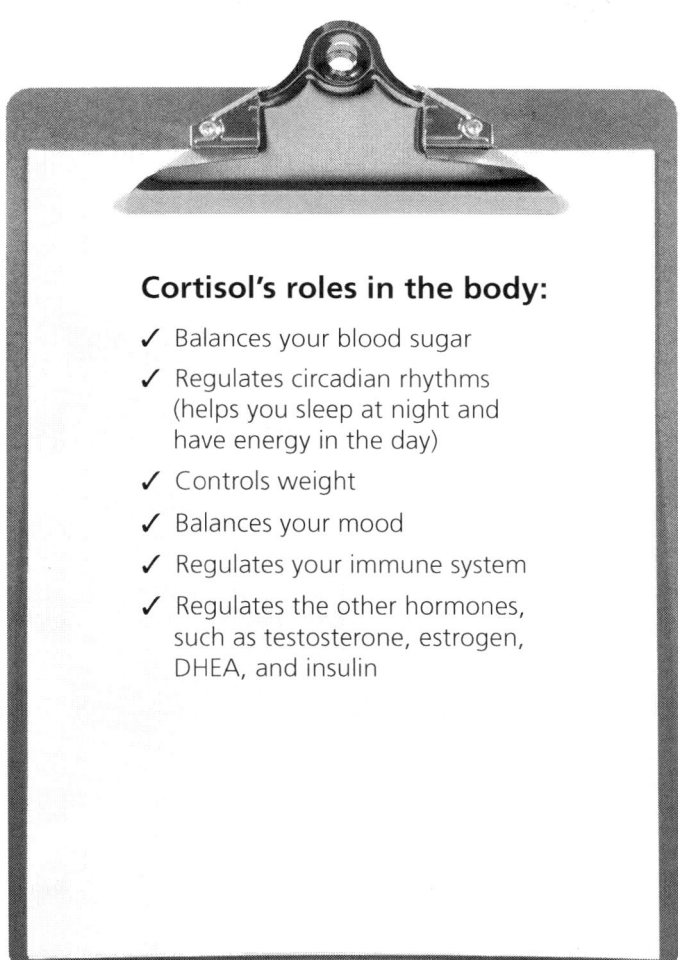

Cortisol's roles in the body:

- ✓ Balances your blood sugar
- ✓ Regulates circadian rhythms (helps you sleep at night and have energy in the day)
- ✓ Controls weight
- ✓ Balances your mood
- ✓ Regulates your immune system
- ✓ Regulates the other hormones, such as testosterone, estrogen, DHEA, and insulin

times of the day. Remember, it's kind of like "long acting adrenaline." Cortisol rises in the wee hours of the morning, kind of like a mini-adrenaline rush, to help you wake up and bounce out of bed (before the alarm goes off) ready to start your day. It gradually declines over the day so you can fall asleep and sleep soundly through the night.

This variation in cortisol release is very important. If you've lost this normal pattern of cortisol release, it's a sign that your HPA axis (the hormone messaging system to help you cope with stress) is malfunctioning.

If you have a blood test done, we'll get a completely different result depending on what time of the day you go. You should have your blood drawn as close to 8 a.m. as possible, because that is the time that the lab uses for its normal range. But there is so much more information that we can learn.

A better test is to collect saliva (2) or urine samples at home at different times of the day.

Your cortisol could be high or low throughout the day, and we could even find that you are too low in the morning (so you're tired during the day) and too high at night (so you can't sleep!). The pattern that we see helps predict what strategy to use to fix the problem.

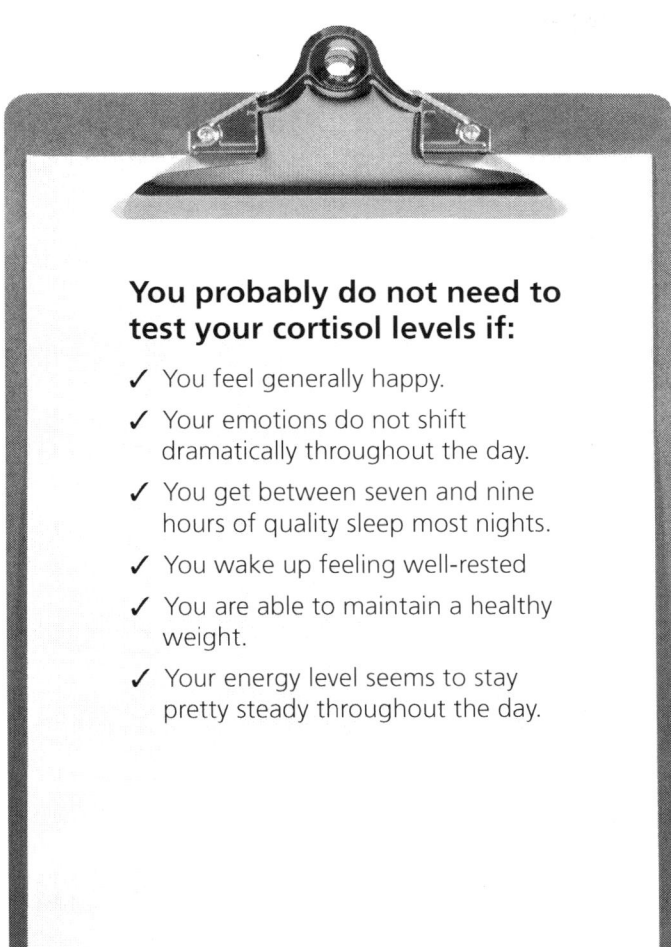

You probably do not need to test your cortisol levels if:

- ✓ You feel generally happy.
- ✓ Your emotions do not shift dramatically throughout the day.
- ✓ You get between seven and nine hours of quality sleep most nights.
- ✓ You wake up feeling well-rested
- ✓ You are able to maintain a healthy weight.
- ✓ Your energy level seems to stay pretty steady throughout the day.

Why Can't I Keep Up Anymore?

Should you go to the trouble of getting a panel of tests?

You probably do not need to test your cortisol levels if:

- You feel generally happy
- Your emotions do not shift dramatically throughout the day
- You get between seven and nine hours of quality sleep most nights
- You wake up feeling well-rested
- You are able to maintain a healthy weight
- Your energy level seems to stay pretty steady throughout the day

On the other hand, you may want to consider testing your hormonal levels with a panel of tests if:

- You struggle with anxiety, depression, or irritability
- You depend on some sort of caffeine to get going and maintain your energy level throughout the day
- You generally don't sleep well and can't remember when you got a full seven hours of sleep
- You can't seem to lose weight, even after trying numerous diets
- You have carbohydrate or sugar cravings, especially when you feel stressed
- You have to drag yourself out of bed in the morning, and have a dip in energy in the afternoon

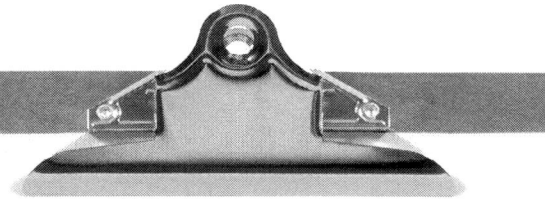

Consider a cortisol test if:

- ✓ You struggle with anxiety, depression or irritability
- ✓ You depend on some sort of caffeine to get going and maintain your energy level throughout the day.
- ✓ You generally don't sleep well and can't remember when you got a full seven hours of sleep.
- ✓ You can't seem to lose weight, even after trying numerous diets.
- ✓ You have carbohydrate or sugar cravings, especially when you feel stressed
- ✓ You have to drag yourself out of bed in the morning, and have a dip in energy in the afternoon

Why Can't I Keep Up Anymore?

What can be done to fix adrenal fatigue?

The first thing is to reduce stress.

Simplify—Are there things you could delegate? Are there things that you could give up (that aren't really that important in the grand scheme of things?)

Don't sweat the small stuff—If you are upset or worried about something, ask yourself, "Will this be important in one year?" If the answer is no, then maybe it isn't worth being upset about.

You may not be able to control all your life circumstances and stresses, but you can control what you choose to think about. If you are a "worrier," and spend a lot of time thinking negative thoughts or ruminating over something that bothers you, you're taking a stressful situation and making it worse.

Instead, try to be an optimist (a "glass half full" person). If things aren't that important, just let them go. By being more positive, you can take that same stressful situation and reduce the effect of stress on your body.

Remember, your brain doesn't know the difference between reality and imagination.

Imagine you are walking down a dark alley, and you are worried that someone is going to jump out and mug you. You are scanning the dark corners, and you're staying on high alert—just in case. Your brain doesn't know that there isn't anyone besides you in that alley, and it is going to send stress signals as though you are really being mugged. The more you worry that a mugging could happen, the more stress signals will be sent.

It's probably wise to be a little "on alert" if you are in a dark alley! But we often do this on a small scale many times a day, and your brain can get stuck in the "on" position and continue to signal for more cortisol to be released—even when nothing stressful is happening!

Training your brain to relax, feel calm, and stop sending stress signals is powerful medicine! I can't give it to you in a pill—it is something that you have to do for yourself.

I can't do your sit ups or eat your broccoli for you either, but you probably know that you should be exercising and eating more vegetables. It is often harder to understand how important it can be to take steps to calm your brain and reduce stress. This really should be a priority if you want to have peak performance and optimal health.

Here are some stress reducing habits that can make a really big difference to your energy, sleep, sex life, belt size, and so much more.

- Breathing exercises
- Meditation
- Visualization
- Yoga
- Tai chi

If these feel like "chores," or you're not quite convinced in the power of meditation yet, here are some other suggestions:

Why Can't I Keep Up Anymore?

- Go for a walk
- Laugh
- Pray
- Be outside in nature
- Pet your dog
- Do something every day that makes you happy
- Try to resolve issues that are causing major stress in your life

Here are some other important things that help reset your stress response:

Eat healthy food

Sugar and the "white stuff" (white flour, potatoes, rice, etc., which spike your blood sugar) stimulate your adrenal gland. We want to give your adrenal system a break!

Instead, go for healthy fruits and veggies that give your hormones the right nutrients to do their job.

Sleep

Try to get to sleep by ten o'clock every night. Why is that the magic hour? If you stay up past 11 p.m., your adrenal glands kick in to help you stay awake. This puts stress on your system and starts a cycle you do not want to continue. Strive for at least eight hours of sleep each night. If you keep your bedtime consistent, your body will eventually get used to the routine and you will feel sleepy around 10 p.m.

Stressed Out

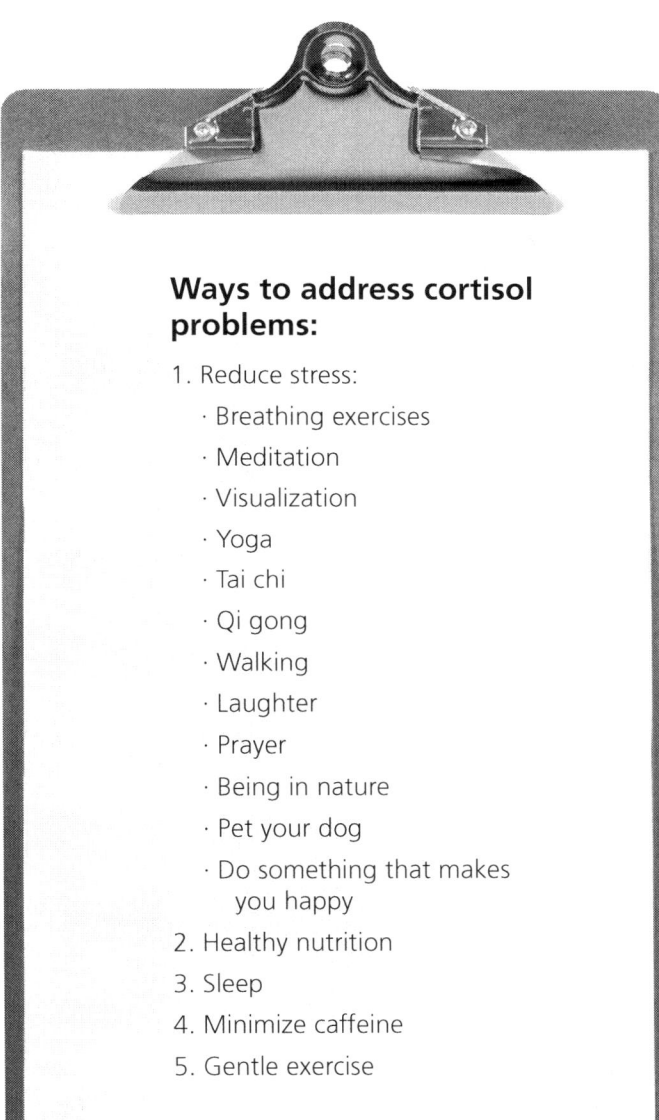

Ways to address cortisol problems:

1. Reduce stress:
   - Breathing exercises
   - Meditation
   - Visualization
   - Yoga
   - Tai chi
   - Qi gong
   - Walking
   - Laughter
   - Prayer
   - Being in nature
   - Pet your dog
   - Do something that makes you happy
2. Healthy nutrition
3. Sleep
4. Minimize caffeine
5. Gentle exercise

Why Can't I Keep Up Anymore?

Minimize caffeine

Try herbal tea instead of caffeinated beverages. Caffeine is a stimulant, and it results in similar effects as stress. It may make you more alert for a few hours, but in the long run it is making things worse.

Exercise

You don't have to go crazy and get a personal trainer with a death wish. Just twenty to thirty minutes most days is great. Try to balance aerobic exercise, strength training (weights), and flexibility.

If you are really exhausted, gentle exercise like yoga or tai chi is best. You should feel better after exercise, not so tired that you want to go home for a nap.

Nutritional supplements for adrenal health

There are a number of herbs that can help support adrenal function—these are known as adaptogenic herbs. They are helpful in resetting the normal circadian release of cortisol (so you make the right amount at the right time of the day).

We now have modern science to understand how they work, but they've been used for thousands of years all over the world to help cope with stress.

Some examples are:

- Rhodiola (3)
- Ashwagandha (4)

- Cordyceps (a type of mushroom)
- Holy Basil (5)
- Ginseng (6)

If your cortisol level is high, a supplement called Phosphatidylserine (7) can help.

How to find help for cortisol problems

As you can see, addressing cortisol levels and HPA axis function is very important for optimal health. If you try to ask your regular doctor for help here, prepare to be disappointed. They simply weren't trained to deal with this problem. They weren't trained to order or interpret the tests (and are likely not aware that anything is even available, other than testing for the life-threatening adrenal diseases). They certainly aren't trained to interpret the results or treat the problem.

You will need to find a Functional Medicine provider to help you resolve the issues. This is so important, because while simple changes in your daily life may make all the difference to your health and well-being, sometimes that is not enough. You may require further tests to look for hidden infections or other hidden issues that may be at the root of your problem, and you'll need a trained Functional Medicine provider to guide you.

CHAPTER 10

5 Steps to Stronger Erections

Many men notice that erectile function changes with age. You may find that your erections are not as strong as they used to be, and you may not always be able to count on your ability to get or maintain an erection.

ED does not necessarily mean that you can't have an erection at all. Erections can be kind of like a bad employee—sometimes they show up, sometimes they don't, and even when they do show up, they don't always do a good job....

Many men associate erections with their identity as a man. When problems occur, you may lose confidence in yourself and in your ability to please your partner. This often triggers depression or anxiety, which can affect more than just the sexual aspects of your relationship. Intimacy helps you feel close to your partner, which helps you weather the tough times together. Even social and work activities can be affected when you aren't feeling good about yourself.

Why Can't I Keep Up Anymore?

This issue may not just be affecting you.

One of my patients, who we'll call Franklin, is typical of many men that I see. He is a 50-year-old man who has been happily married for 20 years. His wife (we'll call her Tina) is a patient of mine. Now that we have her hormones back in balance, she is more interested in sex than ever before. Unfortunately, Franklin's erections are less strong, and he sometimes loses the erection in the middle of intercourse, making the experience unsatisfactory for both of them. Because he worries about his performance, he has become less likely to initiate sex. He hadn't realized how much this was affecting Tina until one day she asked if he found her less attractive. This problem was affecting self-esteem for BOTH of them!

Another patient, Jim, is divorced and is now in a new relationship. He is thrilled with his new partner, who is 10 years younger than him, but embarrassed about his sexual performance. He uses Viagra, which is helping, but doesn't really want her to know. He feels ashamed that he is hiding something from her and wishes that he didn't have to worry or take a pill.

If you aren't currently in a relationship, the lack of confidence triggered by ED can make it harder for you to find someone special.

Problems with performance can be hard to talk about and can feel very isolating. The unfortunate truth is that things tend to get worse with time, so now is the time to do something about it!

5 Steps to Stronger Erections

Don't let ED rob you of confidence and self-esteem. Don't let your life pass you by, or procrastinate and allow the situation to get more dire. There are treatments that can be very effective!

Causes of ED

There are many factors that affect erectile function (for better or worse). And there are many things that you can do to help make things better. But sometimes men are disappointed when they try something, and it doesn't result in improved erections.

Stress (which causes higher cortisol and lower testosterone) also results in less erections. Your nervous system is important to trigger an erection. Stress triggers your sympathetic nervous system "fight or flight" stress response which turns off erections. You need to be relaxed and allow the parasympathetic nervous system to trigger an erection.

Working on stress is important. Reducing stress by simplifying and changing your reaction to stress with meditation and breathing exercises can help.

Anxiety is a big problem with ED. If you are concerned about your performance and your anxiety and stress level go up, then it is more likely that your performance won't be great, reinforcing the problem

Depression often goes along with anxiety and stress and can affect your performance. Many anti-depressant medications are well known to interfere with erectile function. How depressing is that?

Why Can't I Keep Up Anymore?

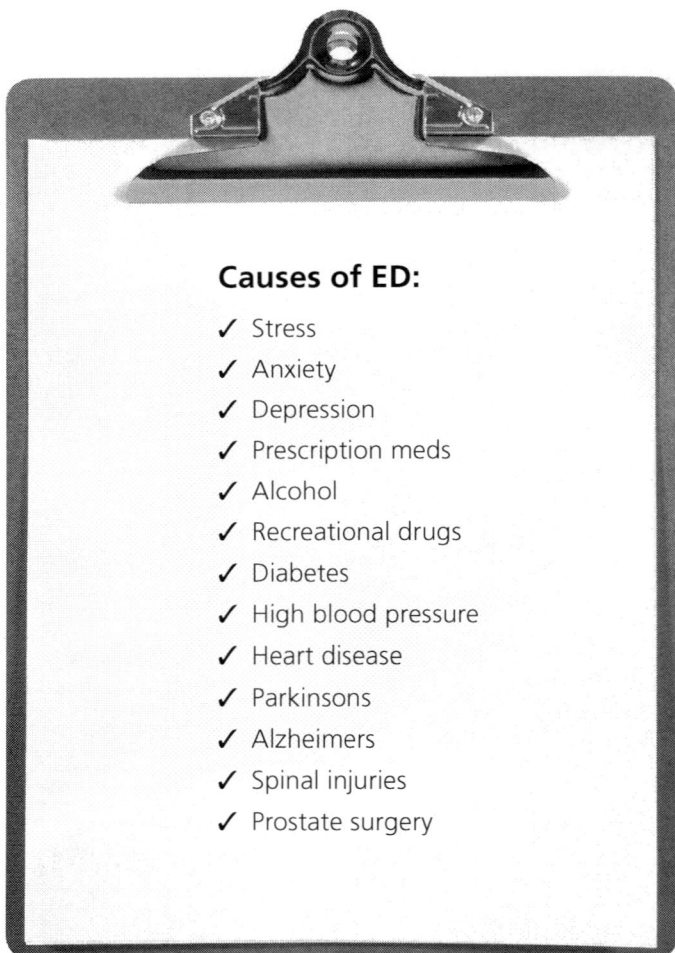

Causes of ED:
- ✓ Stress
- ✓ Anxiety
- ✓ Depression
- ✓ Prescription meds
- ✓ Alcohol
- ✓ Recreational drugs
- ✓ Diabetes
- ✓ High blood pressure
- ✓ Heart disease
- ✓ Parkinsons
- ✓ Alzheimers
- ✓ Spinal injuries
- ✓ Prostate surgery

5 Steps to Stronger Erections

Prescription medications can also cause problems including beta blockers, which are often used for anxiety, heart issues, and high blood pressure.

High blood pressure is a common cause of ED, and ED is a side effect of many blood pressure medications! Double whammy…

Heart disease and ED often occur together. In fact, ED can be an early warning sign of heart problems! If you have plaque in the arteries feeding your heart, you also have plaque in blood vessels everywhere in your body! If blood flow to the penis is reduced due to plaque buildup, you will not be able to have a strong erection.

Diabetes results in both plaque in your blood vessels as well as nerve problems—and both of these contribute to ED. Improving blood sugar control can be very important to help improve erections.

Certain neurological conditions can also result in ED, such as Parkinson's. Nerve damage and spinal cord injuries can cause problems. This type of ED is often more difficult to treat.

The factors that go into creating a strong erection are actually pretty complicated!

Charles Runels, MD suggests thinking about erectile function like a fire.

You may be told that matches are important for a good fire. You strike a match, but there is just a tiny amount of fire, and it only lasts a few seconds, so you decide that matches didn't work.

Why Can't I Keep Up Anymore?

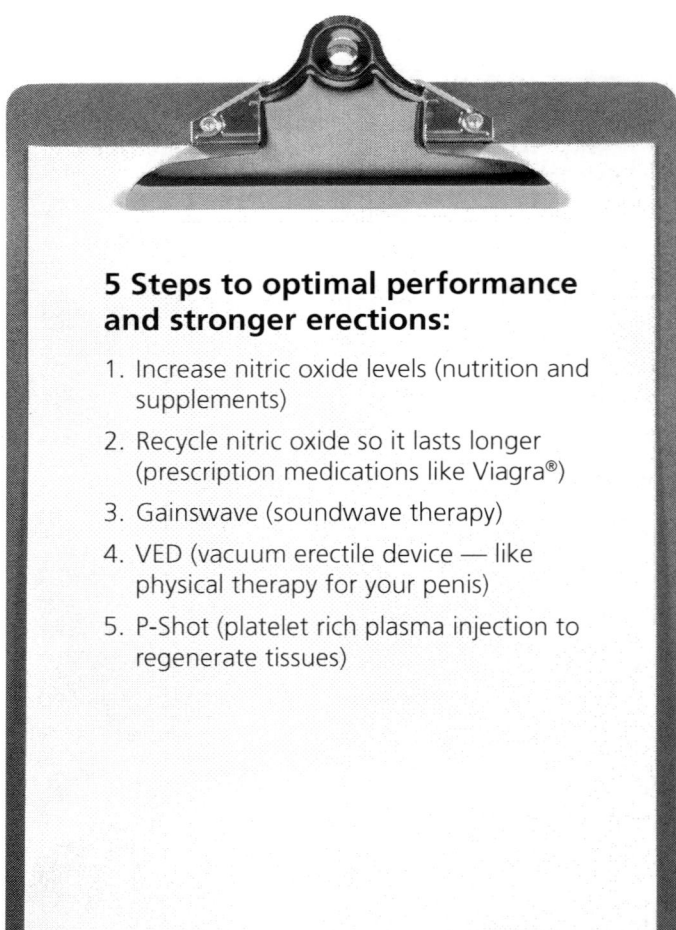

5 Steps to optimal performance and stronger erections:

1. Increase nitric oxide levels (nutrition and supplements)
2. Recycle nitric oxide so it lasts longer (prescription medications like Viagra®)
3. Gainswave (soundwave therapy)
4. VED (vacuum erectile device — like physical therapy for your penis)
5. P-Shot (platelet rich plasma injection to regenerate tissues)

5 Steps to Stronger Erections

Someone else tells you that you need a stack of wood. So, you stack up some wood and wait, but nothing happens so you decide that wood doesn't work.

You hear that lighter fuel can help you with your fire, so you pour some on the ground, but again nothing happens, so you decide that it doesn't work for you.

But if you put lighter fluid on the wood, then light the match, you know what happens!

There are multiple steps that need to happen for you to have and sustain a strong, firm erection. Treatment should target these different areas to get the best results!

On the other hand, there are things that act like water on the fire. These things should be avoided!

Smoking, an unhealthy diet (especially one high in sugar), lack of exercise, and chronic stress all act like water on the fire. In fact, if you are a smoker you should pretty much expect to have erectile dysfunction at some point. Now would be a great time to consider quitting.

The good news is that we have a lot of great options to help! Let's gather the matches, the wood, and the lighter fuel and get started...

5 Steps to Optimal Performance and Stronger Erections

1. Nitric oxide (NO) is the chemical signal that triggers the blood vessels to dilate, or open up, to allow more blood flow to create an erection. (1) When the erection reaches a certain point, the pressure of the blood filling the penis squeezes the

Why Can't I Keep Up Anymore?

veins closed so the blood cannot run out and the erection is maintained. If the erection is not strong enough initially, then the blood will gradually leak out and the erection is lost too soon.

Nitric oxide is key to triggering an erection. Production of NO decreases with age, and with chronic inflammation. Boosting NO is a great way to promote a stronger erection. It is also helpful with blood pressure and heart health....

Certain foods, such as beets, are natural sources of NO. And certain amino acids can also make a difference. Arginine is a naturally occurring amino acid that triggers NO release.(2) It also helps trigger release of HGH, which is the hormone of youth and vitality. Another amino acid, called Citrulline, (3) helps promote the conversion of NO, so a combination of the two often works well. The dose must be high enough to get a benefit. Typically doses of up to 5000mg of Arginine and 1000mg of citrulline are used.

2. Now we've boosted NO. Another option is to keep the NO around longer so it can work harder. This is what sildenafil (Viagra), tadalafil (Cialis) and the other related ED drugs do.

The enzyme phosphodiesterase 5 (PDE5) breaks down NO, and sildenafil is a PDE5 inhibitor, allowing the NO to continue to dilate blood vessels.(4) Of course this is going on everywhere in your body, not just in your penis. So many men complain of headaches (due to dilation of blood vessels in the brain), and other side effects. But if tolerated, it definitely works.

Combining the arginine/citrulline supplement with the prescription medication can increase the effectiveness of the medication, because now there is more NO around for the medicine to work on.(5)

3. Gainswave is revolutionizing performance optimization and treatment of ED.

This is a simple and painless procedure that involves introducing shock waves on the surface of the penis that penetrate and improve blood flow in small blood vessels. (6)(7)(8)(9)(10) The shock waves also stimulate the growth of new blood vessels as part of the body's repair process and bring stem cells (which are the body's natural repair cells) to the area.

Treatments are typically done once or twice weekly for a series of 6-12 treatments. In addition to improved erectile strength, an increase in girth of the penis is often noted.

This is a great treatment for ED in younger men that is caused by stress and anxiety. Since the actual function of the blood vessels of the penis is healthy, the treatment results in strong erections, which help build confidence quickly and overcome the underlying problem. Typically only six treatments are required. For men with underlying health issues like high blood pressure, heart disease or diabetes, at least 12 treatments are recommended.

4. P-Shot is a procedure that can rejuvenate function of the penis. In this simple office procedure, blood is drawn from the

arm (like a regular blood test) and then prepared in a special process to separate out the platelet rich plasma (also called PRP) that contains growth factors. After numbing cream is applied, the PRP is injected into the penis with a tiny needle. The growth factors stimulate the stem cells in the penis to trigger rejuvenation: growth of new blood vessels, nerve endings, and collagen fibers. (11) (12) The effects happen gradually over three months. One treatment can be enough, but often a series of two treatments is done for best results.

5. Vacuum Erectile Devices (VEDs) also make a big difference.

A vacuum device (13) draws blood into the penis to allow more oxygen and nutrients to be derived. If Gainswave treatments and/or a P-Shot has been performed, the pump will help maximize treatment results. It is sort of like physical therapy for your penis—the more you do the stronger erections you will have. Using the pump once or twice daily for 10 minutes will help optimize the results, and then you can do less over the long term to maintain.

Personalizing treatment is important!

Treatment programs can be customized with one or more of these options based on your health history, current issues, and goals.

Young men who don't have ED, but are looking for performance enhancement, will have great results with just a few Gainswave treatments.

5 Steps to Stronger Erections

Older men with more significant ED and underlying medical issues (such as high blood pressure and diabetes) will likely need full treatment with all five of these modalities to see the best results.

Another option: penis injections

For men with more serious erectile dysfunction, there are injections that temporarily increase blood flow and create an erection. The injections typically consist of a combination of medicines including alprostadil, papaverine, and phentolamine, and are called "Trimix injections". The results last for a few hours, so the injection needs to be done each time an erection is desired.

While injecting your own penis may not sound like much fun, the injections are fairly painless and can be quite effective. When nothing else works, it can make a big difference for some men and the small injection may be worthwhile.

Final option—penile implant

In severe cases a penile implant may be considered. This is a surgical procedure where an inflatable rod is inserted into the penis. A pump is hidden in the scrotum. You press the pump to inflate the rod and create an erection. Later you can deflate the rod.

Erectile function and ability to ejaculate are controlled by two different parts of your nervous system. Even if you aren't able to maintain an erection, sensation and ejaculation are usually maintained. An implant can allow penetration, and

Why Can't I Keep Up Anymore?

provide a satisfying experience for you and your partner.

This procedure is not reversible, so it is typically used as a last resort. When all else fails you can have a discussion with a urologist to see if you are a candidate. Even though this is not anyone's first choice, it is nice to know that there are still options even in the worst case scenarios.

CHAPTER 11

Next Steps

Congratulations on being dedicated to taking back control of your health and not being willing to put up feeling less than your best any longer. As you can see, it will require you to be your own advocate and not rely on our healthcare system.

Now that you have learned how things could be different, it's up to you to determine what you will do with the information. Knowledge is not enough. Knowing something will not get you results. Watching the exercise workout on TV while you sit on the couch doesn't get you fit! You actually have to DO something. You need to take action and I encourage you to do just that.

Richard is a patient of mine who decided to DO something. He was a college athlete and a runner but he's 60 now and he's not exercising because life got too busy. He's gained some weight, he tends to snooze in his recliner after dinner, and he has aches and pains that he chalks up to aging. He enjoys his career as an electrical engineer and wants to be able to continue to work and provide for his family.

Why Can't I Keep Up Anymore?

A few years ago, his blood pressure was up, so Richard started on a blood pressure medicine. The next year it was still high, so a second medicine was added. The following year his cholesterol was up. Now he takes Lipitor.

And this year? "Richard, you've got diabetes." In looking back at his labs from the prior years, his doctor could see that his blood sugar level had been going up, but it wasn't even mentioned until it became a serious problem. And what do you think happened next? Another prescription to lower his blood sugar.

Richard was not happy with his state of health. He didn't feel sick, but he certainly didn't feel great. He definitely didn't want to be on all these medicines! When he heard about me from a co-worker he decided to take back control of his health.

Within six months, Richard had lost 50 pounds. His blood sugar and cholesterol are normal—without medicine. He isn't diabetic anymore! He still needs one blood pressure medicine, but his blood pressure is well-controlled. And he feels great! He is even back to running! I don't usually recommend running as the first choice of exercise for a 60 year old, but it is what he loves and he is happy to be able to do it.

If Richard had NOT come to see me, this may have happened instead:

He would have started on the blood sugar medicine, but he still wouldn't be feeling good, so he wouldn't have the energy or motivation to exercise or eat right. He would probably gain more weight, his blood sugar levels would

Next Steps

creep up, and more and more diabetes medicines would be added.

Instead of traveling with his wife, running, and giving back to his community—Richard may have ended up at dialysis three days a week, with a few toes missing due to amputations. Not where anyone would choose to be!

Fortunately, Richard was able to gain control of his health, and give himself a chance for a much better future. And you can, too.

The next step is to find a Functional Medicine practitioner to work with. Here are some tips to help choose the right doctor.

1. I recommend working with someone who is a prescribing medical doctor (an MD or DO, or a nurse practitioner or physician assistant). There are chiropractors and naturopaths and other natural health practitioners out there who can help you improve your nutrition and lifestyle habits, recommend supplements, and start you on the path to feeling better. They can't prescribe testosterone replacement or other prescription medications, however, should those be appropriate.

2. It is also important that your doctor be properly trained in Functional Medicine. There are several places that doctors can go for training, and some are listed below. Your regular doctor may prescribe testosterone replacement, but they will only have a very basic knowledge about how testosterone fits into the big picture, and you may not get the best results.

Why Can't I Keep Up Anymore?

3. Make sure your doctor has experience in treating men's health concerns. Many doctors are turning away from conventional, pharmaceutical medicine because they can see it is not really making their patients well. They are learning about Functional Medicine and opening up private offices, which is great! The more doctors who practice Functional Medicine, the more patients will get well, and the more this process will become standard treatment (which would be wonderful!). But please make sure that the doctor you choose knows what they are doing. You don't really want to be their test case.

4. Make sure the doctor is not a one trick pony. It has become fairly common for men's clinics and hormone pellet clinics to open. They are run by business people who often hire anyone with a medical license and only offer one solution, such as testosterone pellets for example. If only one treatment is recommended, that is a big red flag. They should have a variety of treatment options and should be recommending the best one for you based on your personal health status.

5. The doctor should take time to listen to your concerns and answer all of your questions. You should not feel like you are being herded through the process like cattle. This approach requires more time than a typical doctor's appointment. If you are rushed in and out in only a few minutes, you haven't had a Functional Medicine approach.

6. The doctor should have some personal experience with not feeling well. They may not have the exact same story as you, but they should have some idea of how you feel. When you know something is off, but you're really not sure what it is, how serious it is, how much worse it could get, or if there is even any chance you could feel better—that is not a great place to be. They should have some compassion for your situation, and not blow you off and tell you it's because of your age or that everything is normal. They should dive in, roll their sleeves up and get started on the detective work to figure out where things are going wrong and what needs to be done to fix the problem!

There are doctors like this who are well trained, motivated and ready to help you. Sometimes it can be a little hard to find them, because they aren't working at your local hospital or the large medical clinic in town. They are typically independent doctors, with their own private clinics, and they are great at Functional Medicine (but probably not great at marketing). You may have to do a little work to find someone, but here are a couple of places to look:

American Academy of Anti-Aging Medicine (A4M)

This organization has a training program called the Metabolic Medicine Institute (MMI) which offers a Fellowship in Anti-Aging and Regenerative Medicine (which has more recently been renamed Fellowship in Anti-Aging, Metabolic and Functional Medicine). Doctors who have completed this fellowship will have the letters FAARM behind their name. Some doctors who have taken the extra step to pass an oral board exam (from the American Board of Anti-Aging and Regenerative Medicine) to demonstrate their capability will have the letters ABAARM behind their name.

I have had the privilege to be one of the oral board examiners for almost 10 years. I know the kind of complicated cases that these doctors are asked to address during the exam, and the high level of competency that is required to pass, so I feel comfortable recommending that if you can find a doctor with ABAARM certification, they will know what they are doing.

You can search for a provider at A4M.com. They have a provider directory, so you can look for someone in your area. Be on the lookout for someone with ABAARM certification. If they don't have that certification, it doesn't mean that they aren't an excellent doctor with lots of training and experience, it just means that we don't know.

Institute of Functional Medicine (IFM)

This is another organization which has trained many doctors in Functional Medicine. They also have a Fellowship program, and the practitioners who have successfully graduated and met the requirements will be listed as Institute of Functional Medicine Certified Practitioner (IFMCP).

You can find a practitioner at IFM.org.

Next Steps

Interested in learning more about working with me and my team?

If you are interested in working with us, we would be honored to help you! We work with busy men every day who are looking for real solutions to their health issues.

You can find more information at our website, www.signaturewellness.org. Use the contact us page on our website to schedule a complimentary discovery call with one of our Patient Care Coordinators so we can find out more about you and see if we may be a good fit.

We are in Charlotte, NC, and typically see people locally in our office. We routinely have people drive several hours, or even fly in periodically for appointments. If you live far away, we can do the more advanced testing that your regular doctor doesn't offer, and work with you and your doctor via telemedicine to help optimize your care.

If you want to feel your best, it doesn't have to be hard. You just need to work with the right person who will order the right tests and help you find the right solutions! More energy, a sharp mind, a leaner, stronger body, and great sex are the reward.

Don't procrastinate! You only have one life to live. Don't let it pass you by.

You deserve to live well!

And like I always say, living WELL is the best medicine.

GLOSSARY

5alpha Reductase—A hormone that converts testosterone into estrogen

Adrenal Fatigue—A non-medical term that refers to fatigue resulting from chronic stress

Anastrozole—A prescription medication typically used to block estrogen in women with breast cancer. It may also be used off-label in men to reduce the conversion of testosterone into estrogen

Anti-Aging Medicine—A medical approach that helps to detect, treat and prevent diseases associated with aging

Arginine—An amino acid supplement that dilates blood vessels to enhance blood flow

Ashwagandha—A plant that is typically used to improve the symptoms of stress. Some studies support its use for increasing fertility and testosterone levels in men

Atrazine—An herbicide that can negatively affect reproductive health

Why Can't I Keep Up Anymore?

Autoimmune—A type of health condition that occurs when the immune system attacks part of your own body

Beta-glucuronidase—An enzyme produced in the intestines that breaks the bond between glucuronic acid and toxins, allowing toxins to be reabsorbed into the body instead of excreted in stool

Bifidobacter—Beneficial bacteria included in the gastrointestinal tract. They promote health and can be ingested as probiotics

Calcium Carbonate—A common form of calcium found in dietary supplements

Chrysin—A natural flavonoid that helps reduce the conversion of testosterone into estrogen

Citrulline—A naturally occurring amino acid that is converted to another amino acid called arginine. When taken as a supplement, it may help with erectile dysfunction

Clomiphene—A prescribed medication that stimulates ovulation in women. It may also be used off-label in men to increase testosterone and sperm count

Compounding Pharmacy—These pharmacies fulfill unique prescription orders that cannot be met by a commercially available drug stores

Glossary

Cortisol—The main stress hormone produced by the body's adrenal glands

Cyanocobalamin—A synthetically made form of vitamin B12 that is used to treat vitamin B12 deficiencies and the associated side effects

DHEA—A hormone produced by the body's adrenal glands that is a precursor to sex hormones. DHEA supplements can be used to increase sex drive and muscle strength

DHT—An androgen derived from testosterone. High levels of DHT are linked to hair thinning and male balding

Diabetes—A group of diseases resulting from the body's inability to fully process blood glucose. There are two types of diabetes

Erectile Dysfunction (ED)—a condition when men regularly have problems getting and maintaining an erection

Erythrocytosis—A disorder in which the body produces too many red blood cells, leading to thickened blood and increasing the likelihood of blood clots

Estrogen—The primary female sex hormone. Estradiol and estrone are two forms of estrogen found in men

Why Can't I Keep Up Anymore?

Folic Acid—The synthetic version of folate, both of which are B vitamins

Functional Medicine—A personalized approach that identifies and addresses the root cause of a disease rather than simply treating the symptoms

Gainswave—A treatment for erectile dysfunction that uses sound waves to stimulate blood flow

Gastroesophageal Reflux—Retrograde flow of stomach acid into the esophagus which can irritate the lining of the esophagus

Gynecomastia—Enlargement of male breast tissue often due to sex hormone imbalances

Human Chorionic Gonadotropin (HCG)—A hormone produced by cells that form the placenta in pregnant women. In men, it can be injected to increase the production of testosterone

Human Growth Hormone (HGH)—A hormone produced by the pituitary gland that promotes growth in adolescents and promotes health in adults

Holy Basil—a plant that originates in India and has been used to reduce stress and anxiety

Glossary

HPA Axis—Stands for hypothalamic-pituitary-adrenal axis; it is the central stress response system that, when activated, leads to the release of cortisol

IGF-1—A hormone that stimulates the growth of bone and tissue

Lactobacillus—Genus of bacteria included in the gastrointestinal microbiota. They can be found in food such as yogurt and taken as a dietary supplement

Luteinizing Hormone—A hormone that stimulates production of testosterone in the testes in men

Magnesium Oxide—A common form of magnesium found in nutritional supplements

Microbiome—A collection of microorganisms that inhabit the human body

Nitric Oxide—A molecule produced by the body that is important for blood vessels and good circulation

Omega 3—Fatty acids that can be found naturally in foods such as fish and nuts. Three important forms of omega 3 fatty acids are EPA, DHA, and ALA

Panax Ginseng—A plant whose root is used as a medicine

for various conditions, including helping with stress

Penile Implant- An inflatable rod which is surgically implanted into the penis to treat erectile dysfunction

Penis Pump—A device used to draw blood into the penis to create an erection

Phosphatidylserine—A fatty substance that can be absorbed from diet, produced in the body, or taken orally. It protects cells and aids in cell communication, and may be taken as a nutritional supplement

Pituitary Adenoma—A benign, slow-growing tumor on the pituitary gland

Pituitary Gland—A small gland located under the brain that produces and secretes numerous hormones

Platelet Rich Plasma (PRP)—a concentration of your own platelets, which contain growth factors. PRP injections are used to accelerate healing or regenerate tissues

Primary Hypogonadism—A malfunction of the testes that results in low testosterone and numerous side effects such as low sex drive

Glossary

Probiotics—Microorganisms that have health benefits and can be consumed in foods such as yogurt or dietary supplements

Prolactin—A hormone produced by the pituitary gland that increases breast milk production in pregnant women. In men, high prolactin levels can interfere with testicular function

PSA—Acronym for prostate-specific antigen; high levels of this antigen can be a sign of prostate cancer

P-shot—The process of extracting platelet-rich plasma and injecting it into the penis to promote stronger erections

Rhodiola—A plant whose root is referred to as an "adaptogen." It can be used to help cope with stress and reduce fatigue.

Saw Palmetto—Tree whose fruit is used to decrease negative symptoms of an enlarged prostate and inhibit the conversion of testosterone to DHT

Secondary Hypogonadism—A failure of proper hormone signaling to the testes, resulting in low testosterone levels

Sex Hormone Binding Globulin (SHBG)—A protein produced by the liver that binds and transports testosterone, DHT, and estradiol in the bloodstream, inactivating them from use by the body's tissues

Why Can't I Keep Up Anymore?

Sleep Apnea—A disorder characterized by interruption in breathing during sleep, either from neurological dysfunction or obstruction of airways

Stem Cells—Human cells that have the potential to differentiate into many different type of cells of the body

Testicular Atrophy—shrinkage of the testes

Testosterone Cypionate—An injectable medication given to men who do not produce enough testosterone

Testosterone, Free and Total—The primary male sex hormone that is responsible for male sexual development and reproduction. Free testosterone is not bound to other molecules and is available for use by the body. Total testosterone includes both free testosterone and bound testosterone

Testosterone Pellets—Small pellets containing testosterone that are placed under the skin, releasing testosterone over a period of time

Therapeutic Phlebotomy—The process of removing red blood cells from the body by drawing blood. This procedure is used to treat some diseases

Glossary

Triclosan—An antimicrobial chemical that was used in soaps. The FDA banned its use after failure to prove its safety

Trimix injections—injections into the penis to trigger an erection. Typically a combination of 3 medications (such as alprostadil, papaverine, and phentolamine)

Vacuum Erectile Device (VED)—A device used to draw blood into the penis to create an erection

Vitamin D—A nutrient that can be increased in the body by absorbing sunlight and carries many benefits such as healthier bones

Vitamin E—A nutrient found in foods such as vegetable oils and nuts and behaves like an antioxidant

References

CHAPTER TWO

1. Coates JM, Herbert J. Endogenous steroids and financial risk taking on a London trading floor. Proc Natl Acad Sci U S A. 2008;105(16):6167-6172. doi:10.1073/pnas.0704025105

2. University of Western Ontario, Ivey Business School. "Elevated testosterone causes bull market trading." ScienceDaily, 16 August 2017

3. Newswise 19-May-1998 by University of Utah

4. Wibral M, Dohmen T, Klingmüller D, Weber B, Falk A. Testosterone administration reduces lying in men. PLoS One. 2012;7(10):e46774. doi:10.1371/journal.pone.0046774

5. G. Saad, J.G. Vongas, Organizational Behavior and Human Decision Processes 110 (2009) 80–92

6. Nave G, Nadler A, Dubois D, Zava D, Camerer C, Plassmann H. Single-dose testosterone administration increases men's preference for status goods. Nat Commun. 2018;9(1):2433. Published 2018 Jul 3. doi:10.1038/s41467-018-04923-0

7. Ford AH, Yeap BB, Flicker L, et al. Sex hormones and incident dementia in older men: The health in men study. Psychoneuroendocrinology. 2018;98:139-147. doi:10.1016/j.psyneuen.2018.08.013

8. Hua JT, Hildreth KL, Pelak VS. Effects of Testosterone Therapy on Cognitive Function in Aging: A Systematic Review. Cogn Behav Neurol. 2016;29(3):122–138. doi:10.1097/WNN.0000000000000104

9. Naifar M, Rekik N, Messedi M, et al. Male hypogonadism and metabolic syndrome. Andrologia. 2015;47(5):579-586. doi:10.1111/and.12305

CHAPTER FOUR

1. Emanuele MA, Emanuele NV. Alcohol's effects on male reproduction. Alcohol Health Res World. 1998;22(3):195-201.

2. Cohen PG. Aromatase, adiposity, aging and disease. The hypogonadal-metabolic-atherogenic-disease and aging connection. Med Hypotheses. 2001;56(6):702-708. doi:10.1054/mehy.2000.1169

3. Jannini EA, Screponi E, Carosa E, et al. Lack of sexual activity from erectile dysfunction is associated with a reversible reduction in serum testosterone. Int J Androl. 1999;22(6):385-392. doi:10.1046/j.1365-2605.1999.00196.x

4. Cheung KK, Luk AO, So WY, et al. Testosterone level in men with type 2 diabetes mellitus and related metabolic effects: A review of current evidence. J Diabetes Investig. 2015;6(2):112 123. doi:10.1111/jdi.12288

5. Scinicariello F, Buser MC. Serum Testosterone Concentrations and Urinary Bisphenol A, Benzophenone-3, Triclosan, and Paraben Levels in Male and Female Children and Adolescents: NHANES 2011-2012. Environ Health Perspect. 2016;124(12):1898-1904. doi:10.1289/EHP150

6. Ha M, Zhang P, Li L, Liu: Triclosan Suppresses Testicular Steroidogenesis via the miR-6321/JNK/ Nur77 Cascade. Cell Physiol Biochem 2018;50:2029-2045. doi: 10.1159/000495049

7. Hayes TB, Anderson LL, Beasley VR, et al. Demasculinization

References

and feminization of male gonads by atrazine: consistent effects across vertebrate classes. J Steroid Biochem Mol Biol. 2011;127(1-2):64-73. doi:10.1016/j.jsbmb.2011.03.015

CHAPTER FIVE

1. Vermeulen A, Kaufman JM. Diagnosis of hypogonadism in the aging male. Aging Male. 2002 Sep;5(3):170-6.

2. Bhasin S, Pencina M, Jasuja GK, Travison TG, Coviello A, Orwoll E, Wang PY, Nielson C, Wu F, Tajar A, Labrie F, Vesper H, Zhang A, Ulloor J, Singh R, D'Agostino R, Vasan RS. Reference ranges for testosterone in men generated using liquid chromatography tandem mass spectrometry in a community-based sample of healthy nonobese young men in the Framingham Heart Study and applied to three geographically distinct cohorts. J. Clin. Endocrinol. Metab. 2011 Aug;96(8):2430-9.

3. Jankowska EA, Rozentryt P, Ponikowska B, et al. Circulating estradiol and mortality in men with systolic chronic heart failure. JAMA. 2009;301(18):1892-1901. doi:10.1001/jama.2009.639

4 Schulster M, Bernie AM, Ramasamy R. The role of estradiol in male reproductive function. Asian J Androl. 2016;18(3):435-440. doi:10.4103/1008-682X.173932

CHAPTER SIX

1. Katz DJ, Nabulsi O, Tal R, Mulhall JP. Outcomes of clomiphene citrate treatment in young hypogonadal men. BJU Int. 2012;110(4):573 578. doi:10.1111/j.1464-410X.2011.10702.x

2. Nelles JL, Hu WY, Prins GS. Estrogen action and prostate cancer. Expert Rev Endocrinol Metab. 2011;6(3):437 451. doi:10.1586/eem.11.20

3. Morgentaler A 3rd, Conners WP. Testosterone therapy in men with prostate cancer: literature review, clinical experience, and recommendations. Asian J Androl. 2015;17(2):206 211. doi:10.4103/1008-682X.148067

4. G Corona, G Rastrelli, F Guaraldi, G Tortorici, Y Reismann, A Sforza & M Maggi (2019) An update on heart disease risk associated with testosterone boosting medications, Expert Opinion on Drug Safety, 18:4, 321-332, DOI: 10.1080/14740338.2019.1607290(4)

5. Goodale T, Sadhu A, Petak S, Robbins R. Testosterone and the Heart. Methodist Debakey Cardiovasc J. 2017;13(2):68 72. doi:10.14797/mdcj-13-2-68

6. Morgentaler A, Feibus A, Baum N. Testosterone and cardiovascular disease--the controversy and the facts. Postgrad Med. 2015;127(2):159 165. doi:10.1080/00325481.2015.996111

6. Kloner RA, Carson C 3rd, Dobs A, Kopecky S, Mohler ER 3rd. Testosterone and Cardiovascular Disease. J Am Coll Cardiol. 2016;67(5):545 557. doi:10.1016/j.jacc.2015.12.005(55

7. Snyder PJ, Bhasin S, Cunningham GR, et al. Lessons From the Testosterone Trials. Endocr Rev. 2018;39(3):369 386. doi:10.1210/er.2017-00234

8. Hall, S. American Journal of Cardiology, Jan. 15, 2010; vol 105: pp 192-197.

9. Schulster M, Bernie AM, Ramasamy R. The role of estradiol in male reproductive function. Asian J Androl. 2016;18(3):435 440. doi:10.4103/1008-682X.173932

10. Olsson A, Kopsida E, Sorjonen K, Savic I. Testosterone and estrogen impact social evaluations and vicarious emotions: A double-blind placebo-controlled study. Emotion. 2016;16(4):515 523. doi:10.1037/a0039765

11. Erdemir F, Harbin A, Hellstrom WJ. 5-alpha reductase inhibitors and erectile dysfunction: the connection. J Sex Med. 2008;5(12):2917 2924. doi:10.1111/j.1743-6109.2008.01001.x

12. Ohlander SJ, Varghese B, Pastuszak AW. Erythrocytosis Following Testosterone Therapy. Sex Med Rev. 2018;6(1):77 85. doi:10.1016/j.sxmr.2017.04.001

References

CHAPTER EIGHT

1. Himbert C, Ose J, Delphan M, Ulrich CM. A systematic review of the interrelation between diet- and surgery-induced weight loss and vitamin D status. Nutr Res. 2017;38:13-26. doi:10.1016/j.nutres.2016.12.004

2. Aranow C. Vitamin D and the immune system. J Investig Med. 2011;59(6):881-886. doi: 10.2310/JIM.0b013e31821b8755

3. Garland CF, Garland FC, Gorham ED, et al. The role of vitamin D in cancer prevention. Am J Public Health. 2006;96(2):252-261. doi:10.2105/AJPH.2004.045260

4. Prasad AS, et al. Zinc status and serum testosterone levels of healthy adults. Nutrition. 1996;12(5):344 348. doi:10.1016/s0899-9007(96)80058-x

5. Gerber GS, Kuznetsov D, Johnson BC, Burstein JD. Randomized, double-blind, placebo-controlled trial of saw palmetto in men with lower urinary tract symptoms. Urology. 2001 Dec;58(6):960-4; discussion 964-5. doi: 10.1016/s0090-4295(01)01442-x. PMID: 11744467.

6. Clark JT, Smith ER, Davidson JM. Testosterone is not required for the enhancement of sexual motivation by yohimbine. Physiol Behav. 1985;35(4):517-521. doi:10.1016/0031-9384(85)90133-7

7. Zang ZJ, Tang HF, Tuo Y, et al. Effects of velvet antler polypeptide on sexual behavior and testosterone synthesis in aging male mice. Asian J Androl. 2016;18(4):613-619. doi:10.4103/1008-682X.166435

8. Schöttner M, Gansser D, Spiteller G. Lignans from the roots of Urtica dioica and their metabolites bind to human sex hormone binding globulin (SHBG). Planta Med. 1997;63(6):529-532. doi:10.1055/s-2006-957756

9. Shindel AW, Xin ZC, Lin G, et al. Erectogenic and neurotrophic effects of icariin, a purified extract of horny goat weed (Epimedium spp.) in vitro and in vivo. J Sex Med. 2010;7(4 Pt 1):1518-1528. doi:10.1111/j.1743-6109.2009.01699.x

10. Kamenov Z, Fileva S, Kalinov K, Jannini EA. Evaluation of the efficacy and safety of Tribulus terrestris in male sexual dysfunction-A prospective, randomized, double-blind, placebo-controlled clinical trial. Maturitas. 2017;99:20-26. doi:10.1016/j.maturitas.2017.01.011

11. Rhim HC, Kim MS, Park YJ, Choi WS, Park HK, Kim HG, Kim A, Paick SH. The Potential Role of Arginine Supplements on Erectile Dysfunction: A Systemic Review and Meta-Analysis. J Sex Med. 2019 Feb;16(2):223-234. doi: 10.1016/j.jsxm.2018.12.002. Erratum in: J Sex Med. 2020 Mar;17(3):560. PMID: 30770070.

12. Cormio L, De Siati M, Lorusso F, Selvaggio O, Mirabella L, Sanguedolce F, Carrieri G. Oral L-citrulline supplementation improves erection hardness in men with mild erectile dysfunction. Urology. 2011 Jan;77(1):119-22. doi: 10.1016/j.urology.2010.08.028. PMID: 21195829.

CHAPTER NINE

1. Yaribeygi H, Panahi Y, Sahraei H, Johnston TP, Sahebkar A. The impact of stress on body function: A review. EXCLI J. 2017;16:1057 1072. Published 2017 Jul 21. doi:10.17179/excli2017-480

2. Aardal-Eriksson E, Karlberg BE, Holm AC. Salivary cortisol--an alternative to serum cortisol determinations in dynamic function tests. Clin Chem Lab Med. 1998;36(4):215 222. doi:10.1515/CCLM.1998.037

3. Anghelescu IG, Edwards D, Seifritz E, Kasper S. Stress management and the role of Rhodiola rosea: a review. Int J Psychiatry Clin Pract. 2018;22(4):242 252. doi:10.1080/13651501.2017.1417442

4. Chandrasekhar K, Kapoor J, Anishetty S. A prospective, randomized double-blind, placebo-controlled study of safety and efficacy of a high-concentration full-spectrum extract of ashwagandha root in reducing stress and anxiety in adults. Indian J Psychol Med. 2012;34(3):255 262. doi:10.4103/0253-7176.106022

References

5. Jamshidi N, Cohen MM. The Clinical Efficacy and Safety of Tulsi in Humans: A Systematic Review of the Literature. Evid Based Complement Alternat Med. 2017;2017:9217567. doi:10.1155/2017/9217567

6. Lee S, Rhee DK. Effects of ginseng on stress-related depression, anxiety, and the hypothalamic-pituitary-adrenal axis. J Ginseng Res. 2017;41(4):589 594. doi:10.1016/j.jgr.2017.01.010

7. Hellhammer J, Fries E, Buss C, et al. Effects of soy lecithin phosphatidic acid and phosphatidylserine complex (PAS) on the endocrine and psychological responses to mental stress. Stress. 2004;7(2):119 126. doi:10.1080/10253890410001728379

CHAPTER TEN

1. Cartledge J, Minhas S, Eardley I. The role of nitric oxide in penile erection. Expert Opin Pharmacother. 2001;2(1):95 107. doi:10.1517/14656566.2.1.95

2. Rhim HC, Kim MS, Park YJ, et al. The Potential Role of Arginine Supplements on Erectile Dysfunction: A Systemic Review and Meta-Analysis [published correction appears in J Sex Med. 2020 Mar;17(3):560]. J Sex Med. 2019;16(2):223 234. doi:10.1016/j.jsxm.2018.12.002

3. Cormio L, De Siati M, Lorusso F, et al. Oral L-citrulline supplementation improves erection hardness in men with mild erectile dysfunction. Urology. 2011;77(1):119 122. doi:10.1016/j.urology.2010.08.028

4. Andersson KE. PDE5 inhibitors—pharmacology and clinical applications 20 years after sildenafil discovery. Br J Pharmacol. 2018;175(13):2554 2565. doi:10.1111/bph.14205

5. Gentile V, Antonini G, Antonella Bertozzi M, et al. Effect of propionyl-L-carnitine, L-arginine and nicotinic acid on the efficacy of vardenafil in the treatment of erectile dysfunction in diabetes. Curr Med

Res Opin. 2009;25(9):2223 2228. doi:10.1185/03007990903138416

6. Low-intensity Extracorporeal Shock Wave Treatment Improves Erectile Function: A Systematic Review and Meta-analysis Lu, Zhihua et al. European Urology, Volume 71, Issue 2, 223—233

7. Khodyreva LA, Dudareva AA, Mudraya IS, et al. Efficiency assessment of shock wave therapy in patients with pelvic pain employing harmonic analysis of penile bioimpedance. Bull Exp Biol Med. 2013;155(2):288-292. doi:10.1007/s10517-013-2134-0

8. Srini VS, Reddy RK, Shultz T, Denes B. Low intensity extracorporeal shockwave therapy for erectile dysfunction: a study in an Indian population. Can J Urol. 2015;22(1):7614-7622.

9. Vardi Y, Appel B, Jacob G, Massarwi O, Gruenwald I. Can low-intensity extracorporeal shockwave therapy improve erectile function? A 6-month follow-up pilot study in patients with organic erectile dysfunction. Eur Urol. 2010;58(2):243-248. doi:10.1016/j.eururo.2010.04.004

10. Reisman Y, Hind A, Varaneckas A, Motil I. Initial experience with linear focused shockwave treatment for erectile dysfunction: a 6-month follow-up pilot study. Int J Impot Res. 2015;27(3):108-112. doi:10.1038/ijir.2014.41

11. Epifanova MV, Gvasalia BR, Durashov MA, Artemenko SA. Platelet-Rich Plasma Therapy for Male Sexual Dysfunction: Myth or Reality?. Sex Med Rev. 2020;8(1):106 113. doi:10.1016/j.sxmr.2019.02.002

12. Liu MC, Chang ML, Wang YC, Chen WH, Wu CC, Yeh SD. Revisiting the Regenerative Therapeutic Advances Towards Erectile Dysfunction. Cells. 2020;9(5):E1250. Published 2020 May 19. doi:10.3390/cells9051250

13. Brison D, Seftel A, Sadeghi-Nejad H. The resurgence of the vacuum erection device (VED) for treatment of erectile dysfunction. J Sex Med. 2013;10(4):1124 1135. doi:10.1111/jsm.12046

About the Author

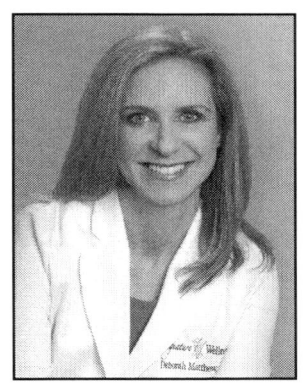

DR. DEB MATTHEW, MD suffered for years with exhaustion and irritability that prevented her from being the wife and mother that she wanted to be. Her quest to resolve her own health issues led her to change everything about her practice of medicine. Instead of just treating diseases with drugs, she helps her patients resolve the root cause of their health issues so they can get well!

With 25 years of clinical experience, Dr Deb works with men and women to help restore their energy, libido, mood and memory.

She is a Diplomat of the American Board of Integrative Medicine (ABOIM) and the American Board of Anti-Aging and Regenerative Medicine (ABAARM). A frequent lecturer for the American Academy of Anti-Aging Medicine (A4M), she has spoken across the US and around the world.

Dr. Deb is a frequent guest expert on national podcasts, radio and broadcast networks including ABC, NBC, CBS, and FOX, and is the best-selling author of *This is Not Normal: A Busy Woman's Guide To Symptoms of Hormone Imbalance.*